T0234691

SpringerBriefs in Public Health

SpringerBriefs in Public Health present concise summaries of cutting-edge research and practical applications from across the entire field of public health, with contributions from medicine, bioethics, health economics, public policy, biostatistics, and sociology.

The focus of the series is to highlight current topics in public health of interest to a global audience, including health care policy; social determinants of health; health issues in developing countries; new research methods; chronic and infectious disease epidemics; and innovative health interventions.

Featuring compact volumes of 50 to 125 pages, the series covers a range of content from professional to academic. Possible volumes in the series may consist of timely reports of state-of-the art analytical techniques, reports from the field, snapshots of hot and/or emerging topics, elaborated theses, literature reviews, and in-depth case studies. Both solicited and unsolicited manuscripts are considered for publication in this series.

Briefs are published as part of Springer's eBook collection, with millions of users worldwide. In addition, Briefs are available for individual print and electronic purchase.
Briefs are characterized by fast, global electronic dissemination, standard publishing contracts, easy-to-use manuscript preparation and formatting guidelines, and expedited production schedules. We aim for publication 8–12 weeks after acceptance.

More information about this series at http://www.springer.com/series/10138

Sarah Cuschieri

To Do or Not to Do a PhD?

Insight and Guidance from a Public Health
PhD Graduate

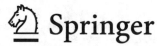 Springer

Sarah Cuschieri
University of Malta
Msida, Malta

ISSN 2192-3698 ISSN 2192-3701 (electronic)
SpringerBriefs in Public Health
ISBN 978-3-030-64670-7 ISBN 978-3-030-64671-4 (eBook)
https://doi.org/10.1007/978-3-030-64671-4

© The Author(s), under exclusive license to Springer Nature Switzerland AG 2021
This work is subject to copyright. All rights are solely and exclusively licensed by the Publisher, whether the whole or part of the material is concerned, specifically the rights of translation, reprinting, reuse of illustrations, recitation, broadcasting, reproduction on microfilms or in any other physical way, and transmission or information storage and retrieval, electronic adaptation, computer software, or by similar or dissimilar methodology now known or hereafter developed.
The use of general descriptive names, registered names, trademarks, service marks, etc. in this publication does not imply, even in the absence of a specific statement, that such names are exempt from the relevant protective laws and regulations and therefore free for general use.
The publisher, the authors, and the editors are safe to assume that the advice and information in this book are believed to be true and accurate at the date of publication. Neither the publisher nor the authors or the editors give a warranty, expressed or implied, with respect to the material contained herein or for any errors or omissions that may have been made. The publisher remains neutral with regard to jurisdictional claims in published maps and institutional affiliations.

This Springer imprint is published by the registered company Springer Nature Switzerland AG
The registered company address is: Gewerbestrasse 11, 6330 Cham, Switzerland

Preface

It all starts and ends with one's ambition and determination, without which one will fail. Having an understandable husband/partner, parents and friends are important ingredients in the life of a doctor of philosophy (PhD) student, spiced up with a supportive supervisor/s. These are all utmost essentials to a successful research career. Along the journey, one would make a lot of acquaintances that may act as assets and be truly helpful but, unfortunately, human nature always precedes and there will be lots of hurdles along the way. There is no straight road or easy shortcut in this research path. This book neither encourages nor discourages someone from reading for a PhD study. It is written to analyse the different aspects of a PhD journey while acting as a guide to those who are about to (or have already) embark(ed) on such a journey, as well as to share personal and colleagues' experiences.

Msida, Malta   Sarah Cuschieri

Acknowledgements

A special thanks goes to my beloved husband who has had my back and shown great moral support and love during the crucial period of my PhD oral defence as well as while writing this book.

Contents

About the Author

Sarah Cuschieri, MD, PhD, MSc, Pg. Dip qualified as a medical doctor in 2011. She studied for a Master of Science degree and Postgraduate Diploma in Diabetes Mellitus Type 2 at Cardiff University in Wales, obtaining a distinction in both between 2012 and 2015. In addition to her Master's degree she was awarded the silver award of excellence by Cardiff University.

After completing her medical training, Dr. Cuschieri took up a full-time academic and research career at the University of Malta in 2013. In 2019, she completed her PhD studies focusing on the "Burden of Diabetes Mellitus Type 2, dysglycaemia and their co-determinants in the adult population of Malta". During the same year (2019), Dr. Cuschieri also obtained a certificate in Public Health Epidemiology at the University of Utrecht in The Netherlands.

A number of Dr. Cuschieri's publications have focused on diabetes mellitus type 2, obesity and medical scientific writing and published in international peer-reviewed journals. Her primary research interests are diabetes mellitus type 2 and obesity and their impact on population health. She has been invited to contribute to a number of book chapters to be published by Springer Nature and Taylor and Francis. Furthermore, Dr. Cuschieri has been invited to be a keynote speaker at international conferences.

Dr. Cuschieri was nominated to join the Military and Hospitaller Order of Saint Lazarus of Jerusalem in 2014 at the Grade of Officer. In 2018, she was promoted to Commander.

In 2018, Dr. Cuschieri co-founded the first NGO targeting obesity in Malta. She currently holds the position of president of the Malta Obesity Association.

Dr. Cuschieri is actively involved in a number of collaborative research projects, particularly in the area of the burden of disease and small member states.

Chapter 1
What Is a PhD? Am I Ready for This Commitment?

The abbreviation 'PhD' stands for Doctor of Philosophy. This is the highest university degree that one can achieve. Those successful in achieving this degree are entitled to use the pre-nominal title of Doctor, with the post-nominal letters such as 'Ph.D', 'PhD' or 'DPhil'. A requisite of this kind of study is to produce an original research that expands the boundaries of knowledge. The subject of the research varies and depends on the student's field of interest or previous studies conducted. In fact, it is customary for the United Kingdom (UK) and European universities to require a Master's degree in the same field of study prior to enrolling in a PhD course. The requirements to earn a PhD degree will vary from one institution to another as well as from one country and another. In the United States (US), PhD students can spend up to a year to evaluate and decide about the research subject they want to follow for their PhD, while attending graduate-level classes. In the US it is also not expected for students to have an in-depth understanding of their research subject right from the start.

Although I achieved my Public Health PhD following a UK-structured PhD programme, references will also be made to other European and US PhD programmes. However, it is important to note that the fundamental principles of a PhD do not vary across countries. Every student will be assigned a supervisor, who is an expert in the research area of interest. The duration of the PhD programme is typically 3 years for full-time and 6 years for part-time students in Europe. For the US, the PhD period may be longer, especially if the student hadn't pursued a master's degree previously. In fact, full-time PhD programmes in the US may take 5–6 years for completion while part-time might take as long as 8–10 years. In the eventuality that a master's degree had been previously achieved, then the duration for completion of the PhD programme would be 4–5 years. At the end of the PhD programme, the submission of a thesis worthy of publication in peer-reviewed journals is expected. Also, students would need to defend their work before a panel of expert examiners appointed by the university.

© The Author(s), under exclusive license to Springer Nature Switzerland AG 2021   1
S. Cuschieri, *To Do or Not to Do a PhD?*, SpringerBriefs in Public Health,
https://doi.org/10.1007/978-3-030-64671-4_1

Why Should I Read for a PhD?

A PhD may not be everybody's cup of tea; however, achieving this degree opens the door to a multitude of career opportunities. It will make your life easier when applying for certain positions. In my case, having an ambitious character I always knew that someday I will embark on this journey. However, it was never on my bucket list to actually read for a PhD so quickly after finishing medical school.

I was faced with a very difficult decision when it was time for me to apply for a basic specialist post (the equivalent of 'Residency' in the US). Having had a working experience in all the different specialities I could envisage myself working as a specialised doctor, I realised that I did not have a real calling for any of the specialities. This created a psychological dilemma. Although I still applied for all the different specialities, I knew deep down I would not be happy. My inner voice was telling me to venture into different pastures. I was blessed that during this period, there was a call for an academic post within the Faculty of Medicine and Surgery at the local university, for which I applied and was awarded the job. This was the perfect opportunity. I was over the moon and delved into a brand new, academic career pathway. Excited as I was, it soon dawned on me that I was faced with a fresh set of challenges—top of which was the fact that I needed to start a PhD programme and finish it within 8 years in order to secure a permanent job at the university. This gave birth to my Public Health PhD journey, which I will refer to throughout the chapters to come.

So as already pointed out, achieving a PhD will provide you with one of the requirements to apply for an academic career, also known as a 'faculty appointment'. However, it is not the sole job opportunity that can be pursued once a Public Health PhD has been achieved. Careers in Science and Research, Healthcare Administration, Directorship in Health divisions, Consultation positions in the private sector, among others, are the most common job opportunities that can be applied for. Remember that once you have achieved your PhD, you would be considered an 'expert' in that field of study. It is imperative to remember that once the PhD is over, you still need to continue your work through research, publications and networking in order to remain on top of the game. When freshly graduated with a doctoral degree, you will be referred to as an 'early career' academic or researcher; this implies that your salary would still be relatively low compared to other colleagues within the same career pathway. However, time and continuous investment in your professional career will help reap financial remuneration in the years to follow.

Some will secure a faculty position as part of their PhD contract (like I did) or others will apply for a faculty position once the PhD is in the bag. Once the PhD has been awarded, you will be awarded a permanent 'Lecturer' position with the faculty you had applied for. This is equivalent to 'Instructor' in the US. This implies that your duties are to teach, supervise and mentor students at your university. In some instances, such as in my case, I also hold a research position apart from an academic one. This means that in addition to teaching, I have to continue researching in my field of expertise as part of my contractual obligations. However, there are faculty appointments that are offered to scientists and scholars to research particular fields as their full-time job. The hierarchy of promotions for both academics and researchers follows the same pathway. Time and effort are the two essential ingredients. Once a lecturer/instructor has distinguished him/herself in his/her respective fields, he/she is eligible for the next promotion, which is 'Senior Lecturer' or 'Assistant Professor' in the United States, followed by 'Associate Professor' and finally 'Professor'. Achieving a 'Professor' title is a testament to the distinguished and exceptional work you had conducted in your field of expertise and elevates your status as an internationally recognised expert. It stands to reason that academic promotions lead to improved financial remuneration.

What Am I Getting Myself into?

Enrolling in a PhD programme is not for the faint-hearted. This is not a walk in the park, but it is a long-term commitment that will change your life. When I was still in the initial thought process behind a PhD (not that I had much of a choice!), one professor told me, 'A PhD is like a marriage; you are stuck with it for at least eight years'. And he was right. Once you take the decision and start the actual research, you will be faced with a number of hardships that you would need to endure. Venturing on such a journey isn't the same as being put on death row; you can run away if it becomes unbearable. But it's obviously a shame to have invested so much time, energy and money and then quit midway.

So, the first question that you need to ask yourself and reflect upon is, 'Do you really want/need to do a PhD?'. It may sound like a simple question, but let me assure you that throughout the course of the PhD programme you will ask yourself this question over and over again. Then again, it is early in this book to come to any conclusions and your perspectives may differ. What I can tell you for now is that there is always a light at the end of the tunnel, irrelevant of how long the tunnel may appear to be. Back to the question at hand, if you are aiming for a faculty career, then you do not have much of a choice; like me, you have to embark on this journey whether you like it or not. The next set of choices would then be crucial in your stage, i.e. where to apply for a PhD (which will be discussed in Chap. 2). On the other hand, if you have no aspirations to get into academia, research, administration or directorship of health care, doing a PhD is not a requisite for your curriculum vitae (CV). Although, to be honest, it is a highly prestigious degree, and you do feel you have achieved an academic endeavour at the end of it. Then again, there are people who consider researching and studying as a hobby. These people are a minority, but I know a professor who did three PhDs; the first was compulsory (for academic purposes), but the other two were done for 'fun'. Personally, I do not think I will go that far. I am ambitious, but not that much!

The second question to consider is, 'Are you ready to adapt your lifestyle?'. Researching, analysing and writing the thesis will take over your life, especially if you are following a full-time PhD programme (shorter duration to complete). In other words, if you are a 9 to 5, Monday to Friday person, you might want to rethink your routine. Your lifestyle will need to be adjusted according to the PhD stage that you are in. On the other hand, you should avoid becoming a slave to your PhD. Your social life and interactions with family, friends and colleagues need to continue. You will need to work out a sustainable timetable that will incorporate both your life and your PhD. There is a possibility that the time spent on 'fun activities' is reduced but not completely decimated.

You need to set priorities in your life. At some point during your PhD journey, working on your PhD will become the priority. Always keep in mind that sacrifices and hard work will pay off at the end. You may be able to complete your PhD earlier than expected, which happened in my case. The following was my jam-packed daily routine. I was following a part-time PhD programme while working full-time as an academic. I was also working a part-time evening job as a medical officer (I was in need of cash); was supervising my house, which was being built and internally finished; as well as planning a wedding. At the time I was juggling all of this on my own since my boyfriend (now husband) was abroad studying and working on his own specialisation. Amidst all this, I still managed to fit in my PhD fieldwork, analyse the data, write the thesis and manage to publish ten publications (all in peer-reviewed international journals). The end result of many sleepless nights—I finished my PhD in 5 years (3 years before the deadline). In other words, the moral of the story is that you can do anything that you set your mind to. It is what you do with your time and the decisions you take that will make or break you. The choice is in your hands; make sure you choose wisely.

The final question to consider is, 'Are you ready to leave the cuckoo's nest and take up a number of responsibilities?'. In most cases, you would need to move close to the university campus, which will entail living costs (housing costs, transportation, health insurance) with a possibility of a student loan. The living costs will vary according to place and country, so it is difficult to define here. As a general rule, staying in a university student's accommodation may be cheaper, especially if you are sharing a place with other students. However, it is something you need to enquire about before coming to a decision. Living close to campus would reduce your transportation costs, but if your research needs to be conducted in different locations or across different institutes this might not be an option for you. It is important to consider the different costs in accordance to your PhD programme and find the best economical solution that suits your needs. Health insurance is a requisite in whichever country you are applying for a PhD. This depends upon your nationality and the country you intend to follow your studies in. For example, an EU/EEA student is automatically covered by the European Health Insurance Card (EHIC) that entitles you to healthcare coverage all across Europe. However, this health insurance is not valid in the US. It is therefore essential that when applying for a PhD programme you make sure that your health insurance is up to scratch; if not, seek help in this regard. All of these factors are additional costs even before you consider the actual university fees. Not everyone is fortunate to be able to self-fund or get a scholarship that will cover all of these costs. Some students would need to either get a part-time job in the vicinity of the campus or obtain a student loan in order to fund the living costs and/or the university fees. This is an additional hardship and commitment that the student needs to consider when applying for a PhD. It is important to remember that such choices are a long-term commitment, especially if you are considering a student loan.

What Types of PhDs Are Out There?

The type of PhD programme a student can follow varies. A student can choose to follow a full-time, part-time, distance-learning/online or hybrid programme. There are also the Joint PhD, PhD by publication and DrPH to consider.

A *full-time PhD* programme will take approximately 3–4 years for European students or 4–5 years for US students to complete. The student will attend the university campus daily, may have an office and will use the facilities provided by the university including the library, technicians, secretaries and many other support staff who will assist the student. The student will also have one or two supervisors who will facilitate the student's research. From the university's perspective, all of these facilities cost money and hence the full-time programme fee will be of a substantial amount.

A *part-time PhD* programme will take a longer time to complete, but the student does not have to study on a full-time basis. In fact, such students can work or be involved in other activities outside the university's life. In such cases, the student will use the university's facilities less often, and consequently the fees are usually a fraction of the cost of those for full-time students. The majority of universities offer this type of PhD programme but usually in limited numbers. Statistically those following a part-time programme have reduced access to university facilities and staff, have distractions from their work and are more likely to lose motivation and direction after so many years. Nevertheless, from personal experience, if the student sets his/her goal to achieve this degree, irrelevant of any part-time hurdles, the PhD can still be achieved.

Distance-learning/online PhD programmes are offered by some universities. In such cases, the student does not have to be physically on campus or in the country for that matter. Teachings, meetings with faculty and all communications will be performed through electronic means. Although this may sound appealing, being away from faculty may lead to difficulties, especially if your research journey becomes bumpy. Obviously, following such a programme would entail lower university fees.

A *hybrid PhD* programme offers a bit of both worlds; i.e. it integrates online and campus-based research and modules. This provides students with the convenience and flexibility of distance learning but also with classroom interactions. Such a programme provides several potential advantages for those students who have to work, as well as reduce the amount of commuting time the student has to endure to the university campus. The duration of this type of PhD programme will generally not differ much from that of full-time programmes; however, it all depends on how efficient the student is in completing the requirements.

Another type of PhD programme is a *joint PhD*, where the student is registered with two universities at once. The idea behind this type of PhD is to strengthen the research collaboration; however, it may not be an easy option. The student will have two supervisors, one from each university. This could lead to potential conflict between the supervisors themselves on any particular topic. Also, the student may feel isolated and not part of a PhD cohort since the research is divided between two institutions. Although joint PhD students have access to training opportunities in both universities, it does not necessarily mean that joint PhDs are an easier way to secure funding. Nevertheless, joint PhDs may result in prestigious collaborations since the student will have access to top researchers in the area of interest. This experience may provide excellent opportunities for PhD students to distinguish themselves from other students.

There are some universities that award a *PhD through publication*. This is not to be confused with the inclusion of publications as a chapter of the PhD thesis. A PhD through publication is awarded to someone who has several publications on a related topic that constitutes a portfolio of original work at a PhD level. The duration of this type of PhD is much shorter since the exceptional research has already been completed and published. All that is required from the student is a coherent body of work with an introduction and a conclusion. The completion of this PhD by publication typically takes around 1 year. A supervisor is usually involved, who will guide the student through the formulation of the thesis. The eligible publications for this type of PhD will vary from academic papers, book chapters, monographs, books, and scholarly editions of text, technical reports, media presentations and surveys. Nonetheless the potential student needs to identify a university that accepts such a PhD type as well as discuss the type of publications that are recognised for such an award.

A *DrPH* programme leads to a doctoral-level qualification that is intended for leaders and future leaders in public health. The aim of such a programme is to equip the student with experiences to deal with challenges as well as adopt scientific knowledge to achieve public health gains. Furthermore, it provides the student with analytical and practical skills required to be managers and leaders in public health. Hence, the DrPH has a dual focus: (1) to develop expertise in the conduction and evaluation of research, and (2) to develop the crucial skills required for leadership roles in public health policy and practice. DrPH programmes mainly focus on general public health, public health practice, health policy and management. On the other hand, public health PhD programmes focus on epidemiology, behavioural science, biostatistics as well as health policy and management. The entry requirements for the DrPH are very similar to those of a PhD, although the student will be required to have experience in areas of public health policy, management and/or leadership. This type of programme is usually offered by public health departments/schools within certain universities.

So, in a nutshell, a PhD in Public Health will prepare the student with the skills needed to make scholarly, research-based contributions to the field of study. This programme will provide the student with the opportunity to contribute to the field through an original dissertation. A number of careers can be pursued following the achievement of a PhD in Public Health including: Epidemiologist, Public Health researcher, Faculty/professor, Postdoctoral fellow, Biostatistician, Global health professional/consultant, Public Health consultant and Public Health policy advisor. On the other hand, a DrPH will open the doors for Public Health leaders, Public Health managers/directors and Health policy-makers.

Chapter 2
The Initial Steps Towards a PhD

When applying for a PhD, it is important to make sure that the university offers the graduate programme in your subject area. It is useless applying to a particular university when it does not accommodate your research area, the training required and the facilities to conduct your PhD research.

Getting a PhD in the United States

There are two major university categories in the United States: public and private universities. Public universities form part of the state university system and receive funding from the state. Hence, these universities will charge local or 'in-state' students less than 'out-of-state' students. On the other hand, private universities do not receive any state funding, so their income depends solely upon the students' fees. Therefore, these students tend to be subjected to higher fees than those that attend a public university. This is usually a flat rate that is kept the same for in−/out-of-state and international students. Apart from the fees, there aren't any concrete differences between the programmes offered by the public and the private universities.

Public universities charge an average of US$13,000 per year for in-state students, while out-of-state and international students are subject to higher annual fees. Private universities charge an average of US$43,000 per year for all students. Fees vary from one university to another, so it is essential to check the fees on the university's website for better clarification.

When choosing the US as the base for your PhD programme, it is important to apply to an accredited university. The 'Council on Education for Public Health (CEPH)' ascertains the quality of public health education and training within the US. Degree programmes and universities offering public health programmes apply to the CEPH in order to achieve accreditation. The CEPH evalu-

© The Author(s), under exclusive license to Springer Nature Switzerland AG 2021
S. Cuschieri, *To Do or Not to Do a PhD?*, SpringerBriefs in Public Health,
https://doi.org/10.1007/978-3-030-64671-4_2

ates each degree programme to ensure that the quality of the programme and the curricula offered reach a satisfactory level. The CEPH gives accreditation through three different categories: schools of public health (SPH), public health programmes (PHP) and stand-alone baccalaureate programmes (SBP). The actual category is irrelevant as long as the actual programme has been accredited. The difference in these categories lies in the extent of options being offered, in which the SPH typically offers a wider range of different degree options than the other categories. In fact, the SPH must offer both a master's degree and a doctoral degree while the PHP and the SBP are free to offer one or more type of degrees. For more information, it is recommended to visit the official CEPH website (https://ceph.org).

Finally, remember that you are going to spend 4–6 years at the university, which is a long time. It is therefore recommended to consider extracurricular factors as well as job opportunities (should you be working part-time to finance your PhD) when choosing a PhD programme. Your work-life balance is an important component to your PhD success.

US Entry Requirements

Universities in the US use a 'Grade Point Average (GPA)' system that measures the academic performance of a student. The GPA considers all the individual academic assessments that a student has completed as part of a degree. A GPA equivalent may be calculated based on the final grades and transcripts the student has achieved. As a rule of thumb, a GPA of 3.0 or higher is 'good enough' for admission to a PhD programme.

Apart from the GPA score, most US universities set up entry exams. These exams assess the student's skill in literacy, numeracy, critical thinking and different types of reasoning. Scoring well in these exams demonstrates the student's academic capability to advance to graduate-level work. Furthermore, if the English language is not the first or native language of the student, then the student needs to sit for a recognised English language test, such as 'International English Language Test System' (IELTS) or 'Test of English as a Foreign Language' (TOEFL). Ultimately, students may be asked to attend an interview prior to being awarded a place in a PhD programme, especially for very competitive PhD programmes.

There are three potential outcomes for a PhD application in the US: (1) successful, (2) unsuccessful, or (3) on the waiting list as a second-choice candidate. Should the first-choice candidate decline the offer or does not enrol in the programme, then the second-choice candidate is offered the place.

Student Visas

It is mandatory for international students to apply for a visa in order to study in the US, unless the student is a citizen of Canada or Bermuda. All other international students will need an 'F Student Visa', which enables the student to study in all academic institutions within the US. In order to apply, the student needs to have been accepted already to study in an accredited university, as well as satisfied the requirements that the student is of good character and is a genuine student. The visa application process is a detailed and lengthy process. It needs to be prepared way in advance of the initiation of the graduate programme itself.

The US PhD Programme

The fundamental pillars of a PhD programme in the United States are different from those of the United Kingdom and continental Europe. The US graduate programme takes longer to complete than that of the UK. Unlike the UK, a PhD student in the US is given time to understand the research subject before focusing on the dissertation proposal. This stage can be referred to as the 'coursework stage'. The student needs to attend a number of taught classes or coursework modules that cover key concepts and research techniques that are required later on for the PhD research. The classes are divided into: (1) core classes—these are essential requirements as part of the graduate programme; however, there are also (2) elective classes—the student would need to complete enough of these classes to satisfy the credits required in accordance with the graduate programme. The good thing about these elective classes is that the student is free to choose whichever topic he/she prefers. Once the classes have been successfully completed, the student then needs to undergo a comprehensive exam, also known as the 'dissertation qualifying exam'. It is only after passing this exam that the student is allowed to start the dissertation research.

Once successful, a research topic needs to be identified and put forward in a dissertation prospectus. This consists of an essay outlining what the student intends to do; i.e. the study design, methodology and the expected outcome along with the relevant literature review. There are some graduate programmes that require the student to present the prospectus and defend the ideas and techniques being presented. A successful prospectus will result in the assignment of a committee of supervisors (a.k.a., advisors) whose expertise and interests align with the research topic at hand. From this point forward, the PhD will follow the same conventional research doctorate as that of the rest of the world.

Getting a PhD in the United Kingdom

The British Government's Quality Assurance Agency for Higher Education (QAA) is responsible for the rigorous assessment of all UK universities. It ensures that the quality of the teaching is exceptional and equal among all universities. The QAA assessment looks into the curriculum design, assessments, learning resources, facilities and student supports offered by each university. Ultimately each course is given a rating out of a total of 24, with anything over 22 considered as 'Excellent'. Hence, students applying for a particular programme within the United Kingdom need to take this score into consideration. There is also another 'research excellence framework' that needs to be considered which focuses on the strength of the research activity of the university's department of interest and is rated on a scale of 'Unclassified to 4*'.

UK Entry Requirements

The entry requirements differ between each graduate programme; however, the higher the ranking of the university, the more stringent the entry requirements will be. It is customary in the UK that as part of the PhD application requirements, the student must have achieved a Master's degree in addition to the undergraduate degree within the same field of study from a recognised university. In addition, international students are required to have a substantial grasp of the English language, which is assessed through the International English Language Testing System (IELTS). IELTS is a popular English language proficiency test through which the student is assessed on listening, reading, writing and speaking skills. When applying for a PhD, the required IELTS score usually ranges between 6.0 and 7.0, although different universities will have different requirements.

The UK PhD Application

Many UK universities strongly advise students to identify and contact a potential supervisor working within the desired university before making a formal application. The potential supervisor needs to be an expert in the chosen field of study. The supervisor will be able to give the student advice and critical feedback on the research idea that will enhance the proposal. This comes in handy as it is often crucial for the proposal to be competitive and well-structured, especially when applying for funding. If, on the other hand, a student is interested in joining an existing research project or research group, a supervisor already would be allocated for this project. Contacting the group/project supervisor of the research will allow the student to identify if there is an opening for a new PhD student to join the existing project as well as to obtain more details about the project.

Universities tend to organise 'open days' for potential students to visit the campus and find out more information about the facilities and programmes offered. During this visit, the student also would be able to meet the academic and administrative staff running a particular faculty or programme. Open days are usually organised once a year, so it is important that students take advantage of these occasions if considering a PhD in the foreseeable future.

University fees will vary depending on whether the student is a full-timer or a part-timer as well as whether the student is a UK/EU resident or an international student. On average, a full-time UK/EU PhD student will pay £5000 per year, while an international student will pay £19,000 per year. For a part-time PhD, UK/EU students will pay an average of £2500 and international students will pay £9500. These fees vary by university as well as by year. The fees usually cover the cost of the graduate programme including registration, tuition, supervision, exams and graduation. The fees also usually entitle the student to access the university's library and resources.

Once a student has chosen the university and PhD programme, then an online application form needs to be completed. A number of documents will be required including a detailed CV, recommendation letters from previous professors and a detailed proposal of the intended research (this does not apply for those applying for an already established research programme). Another factor to remember is that international students (i.e. non-EU) may require a student visa. It is recommended to check with the university prior to applying.

Getting a PhD in Europe

The majority of the PhD programmes in Europe follow the same format. For this section, the structure of The Netherlands PhD programmes will be described.

The research programme follows the same format as that of the UK, where research is carried out on a specific topic and is documented in the form of a thesis, which is defended at the end of the programme. It is customary in The Netherlands (and may differ in other European countries) that PhD students will hold the title of 'professional researchers' and will therefore be paid a salary during their studies. However, the student would be expected to fulfil various duties as a researcher as well as contribute to the university's academic work. These usually involve teaching as well as other responsibilities. It is the responsibility of the individual university to ensure that the quality and the content of the PhD programmes is up to par. The accreditation organisation oversees the quality assurance.

The minimum duration of the typical PhD programme is 4 years. PhD students would be assigned to a supervisor who will oversee the student's research and thesis writing. It is expected that the student publishes at least part of the thesis prior to submission and examination. The unique aspect of following a Dutch PhD programme is that at the end, the defence examination takes the form of a ceremony. All of the examining academics and the student are required to wear traditional academic attire and the defence would follow a formal proceeding.

Considering that the student will be working as part of the PhD programme, the university does not charge the traditional tuition fees. However, there are other types of PhD students who still follow a graduate programme but either would be sponsored by an external source such as a scholarship or are self-funded and will work on the PhD research in their free time. Irrelevant of type of PhD student, all students are required to pay 'statutory fees'. These cover supplementary costs including supervision, examination, administration and university access. The specific amount of the expense will vary from one university to another.

Entry Requirements

The entry requirements typically follow that of the UK, where the student is required to hold a Master's degree in the research subject that originates from an accredited university. Most PhD programmes in The Netherlands are taught in English and hence non-native English speakers will need to undergo English language tests (as described earlier in the chapter). Entry visa and resident permits are required for international students (not applicable for those with EU/EEA or Swiss national status). The application process is typically the same as the one described for the UK.

Chapter 3
Proposal, Permissions and Funding

The Proposal

A PhD research proposal is required by the university either at the very beginning (typically for a UK or European university) or after completion of the coursework stage in the US. Alas, the backbone of a research proposal follows the same structure; i.e. background (literature review), aim and objectives, methodology and expected outcomes. An exceptionally good proposal is not only a winning ticket to enrol in your desired PhD programme but also to secure funding.

The first step you need to take is to identify the subject of your choice, which in my case was 'type 2 diabetes'. This is followed by the decision as to which department you want to apply to. Considering that I am a people's person and following the fact that I wanted to conduct research that would be relevant to my country, it was a no-brainer that the department of Public Health was my number one choice. The next step will vary depending on the country and the university you want to apply for your PhD (see Chap. 2 for more details). It also varies by whether you want to follow a PhD where you choose your own topic (like I did) or else join an existing research centre or project. The latter option will have a pre-defined aim, objectives, research design, expected outcomes, targets and potentially even funding. This kind of PhD will not be described since it all depends on the structural programme and pre-existing guidelines that are specific for each project. However, I will discuss the former type of PhD, where you as the student, will need to choose your own topic, potentially your own supervisor and prepare an original research proposal.

© The Author(s), under exclusive license to Springer Nature Switzerland AG 2021
S. Cuschieri, *To Do or Not to Do a PhD?*, SpringerBriefs in Public Health,
https://doi.org/10.1007/978-3-030-64671-4_3

The Background, Aim and Objectives

Once you have decided on the subject (e.g. type 2 diabetes) and the area of study (e.g. Epidemiology/Public Health), then you need to carry out an extensive and comprehensive literature review. It is important to gain profound knowledge on your subject area and any related matters. This literature review needs to cover local as well as international data in order to identify a potential niche that you can explore further. Once you have a grasp of the subject and its associated literature, it is time to seek expert help; i.e. approach a potential supervisor (unless you have already been assigned one). Ideally the supervisor is an expert in the subject area and obviously is in a position to take on a PhD student. The next step would be to discuss ideas with your supervisor. You will be amazed at how your views and ideas may change once you have had a heart-to-heart discussion with your supervisor. I still remember my first three-hour meeting with my own supervisor. I went in with one idea, which according to me, at the time, was flawless, to come out from that meeting with a totally different idea and a new reading list at hand. So do not feel disheartened if it happens to you too. The reason being, upon speaking with an expert in the field, you will uncover certain niches that you might not have been aware of, or else did not consider it as a niche worthy of investing. In my case, local national data on the health status of the population was long overdue due to lack of research indicators and funding. Considering that type 2 diabetes had long been declared to be the national disease of my country, conducting a national study covering 'type 2 diabetes, the related co-determinants and their metabolic and genetic interactions' presented the perfect aim and objectives for my PhD. Obviously, each country, region, and state will have different public health needs, so again I stress that you need to discuss and approach experts in your subject field. When writing your proposal, the relevant background literature leading to your aim and objectives need to be clearly stated. You need to have a very strong argument as to why your proposed study and hence your research question is relevant and why it should be given the light of day.

The Study Design (Methodology)

Identifying the best study design (methodology) that will enable you to answer your research question is an absolute requisite. There are various study designs ranging from observational to experimental studies. The latter is a highly unlikely choice for a PhD study since it is expensive to conduct and requires a long duration (usually beyond a PhD timeframe) to come to a conclusive result. Observational study designs are more appropriate for PhD research questions. Establishing the correct study design requires epidemiological knowledge, and this is an area that your supervisor can advise you on. In my case, I wanted to assess the health status of my country's population at a particular period of time; i.e. take a snapshot of the health

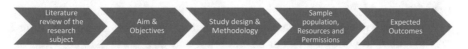

Fig. 3.1 Step-by-step diagram of the proposal components and sections

status. Therefore, the most appropriate study design was a 'cross-sectional study'. This is a common study design followed by public health PhD students (a detailed account of this design will be provided in Chap. 4). Another common study design is a case-control study.

Once the study design is established, you are then in a position to work out your sample population, quantify the material and resources required along with the permissions that accompany it. At this stage, you might need the expertise of a supervisor. The study design along with the detailed resources and permissions required need to be noted in your proposal.

Expected Outcomes

The last section of the proposal needs to list the expected outcomes that you are anticipating from your study. This will be based on the literature you have read as well as the aim and objectives that you have set out to investigate.

This brings us to the end of the proposal. A summary of the different steps and components that need to be included in the proposal are illustrated in Fig. 3.1.

Permissions

Permissions to conduct your proposed study will vary depending on the expected study population, the methodology proposed, the characteristics of the population and the facilities required, among other things. I will discuss the permissions I had to obtain in order to conduct a national cross-sectional study.

If the proposed study design involves direct interaction with human subjects (this also applies for animals), you need to obtain ethics clearance. There are various ethics committees set up; usually there is a university-specific appointed ethics committee that evaluates the research proposals of students studying at the university. If this is not available, enquire about other reputable ethics boards. Every university will have a different ethics structure. In my case, we have a 'Research Ethics Committee' for each faculty that reviews the proposal, materials to be used for the research (e.g. questionnaires, consent forms, information booklets, etc.) as well as reviews a copy of any permissions that were required. The student is invited for an interview with the ethics board to 'defend' the research proposal. If the study is clear-cut and there is no ethical concern, then the student will be given the green light. If the ethics board identifies a potential ethical concern, then the case will move on to the main university's research and ethics committee. In my case, since I was planning to perform a health examination and take blood samples from the study population, it was expected that apart from being grilled by the faculty ethics committee, my proposal would be passed on to the main university's research and ethics committee.

The General Data Protection Regulation (GDPR) is another issue that needs to be tackled if human subjects are part of your study. This is to ensure that the privacy of participants is safeguarded. The process to obtain GDPR clearance for your study will vary by country, region and state. The ethics committee itself may provide GDPR clearance. If not, you will need to apply through another relevant entity. It is important to enquire about this procedure and obtain GDPR clearance. Some general tips on how to comply with GDPR: make sure that the personal details are kept safely and securely by one person—it could be you, as the student, or your supervisor. A unique code is given to each participant that is noted throughout the entire study. Only the entrusted person holding the personal details is able to cross-link the gathered data to the personal data. The personal details can be retained up to a specified period of time only, usually around 10 years, after which the details need to be destroyed securely. How GDPR is being protected throughout the study must be written down on the consent form. The consent form is a letter given to each participant to read, understand and sign as an agreement to participate in your study.

The remaining permissions will depend on your research protocol and methodology. Let's use my example. The random sample population was obtained from a national register; as a result, permission from the government's data protection commissioner was needed. The participants were going to be offered a health examination and have some blood samples drawn in peripheral clinics owned by the Ministry of Health. Hence, permissions and clearances were obtained from the Minster of Health, the Chief Medical Officer, Director of Primary Health as well as Head of Primary Health Care in order to utilise these clinics. The biochemical blood samples withdrawn during the fieldwork were to be analysed by the state's hospital biochemical laboratory at a specified overtime rate. Therefore, permissions from the chairman of the pathology department, the head of the biochemical laboratory and the CEO of the hospital had to be obtained. Since the biochemical blood results were to be accessed through the hospital's online system, data protection clearance from the hospital's data protection unit needed to be secured as well. Apart from this, genetic testing was also anticipated, which necessitated clearance to use the university's genetic laboratory facilities from the director of the biobanking and genetics unit as well as the head of the genetics laboratory.

As you can see there are a number of different permissions and clearances that need to be considered and obtained. It is essential to make a list of potential permissions required together with your supervisor and start tackling them one by one.

Funding

Funding can be divided into two main sections: (1) funding of your PhD studies (university's fees) and (2) funding of the tangible and non-tangible costs of your research.

Funding of the University's Tuition Fees

A. Funding in the US: Some PhD students will be eligible for stipends provided by their institution through an assistantship position (teaching, researching or administrative assistant positions). Other students would need to find their own funding through schemes. The American government offers schemes for student funding such as the 'Fulbright Program' (https://eca.state.gov/fulbright). Furthermore, some universities will provide scholarships for their graduate students. These can vary from 'full' scholarships that will cover tuition fees, living costs and other expenses or 'partial' fee discounts or full fee waivers.

B. Funding in the UK and Europe: This can take three funding routes. The first is self-funding, where the student is responsible for paying their own tuition fees to complete the PhD. The second is to obtain a studentship, where the university would utilise funding obtained from industry partners, research councils or charities to fund research projects. If the student applies for a PhD as part of one of these projects, then the tuition fees are usually covered with a possibility of receiving money for living costs. The last option is to secure a scholarship. There are various entities such as the university itself, the government or third-party research organisations that offer scholarships. An example is the 'Commonwealth scholarships' (http://cscuk.dfid.gov.uk/apply/) that any student originating from a commonwealth country is eligible to apply (terms and conditions apply).

Funding for Your Research Project

This is a crucial step and should not to be taken lightly since without adequate funding your research project will never become a reality. The following section will describe the process of budgeting for your research project, how to formulate a funding proposal and ways of obtaining funding. It is important to note that not every student will be required to do this, since some PhDs have an already established research budget or else are part of the PhD scholarship.

The first step is to formulate an itemised budget for your research project by quantifying and costing all tangible and non-tangible expenses. You need to go step by step through your methodological protocol and cost everything from the stationery used for your questionnaire, to the pen you need to write with, as well as include the salary of any personnel involved in the data collection and analysis. At least three quotes are needed from potential suppliers for the tangible costs, which include consumables and equipment. Once the budget has been compiled then you need to formulate a proposal (very similar to the PhD proposal described previously) that will be presented to the potential sponsors or used to apply for grants or scholarships. The grant proposal is summarised in Fig. 3.2.

A Gantt chart may be required, especially if you are going to present your proposal and budget to potential sponsors. The Generalized Activity Normalization Timetable (GANTT) is a horizontal bar chart that provides a graphical illustration of your planned research schedule. It will give you and the sponsor a timeline—a rough idea of when you will be starting, for example, the fieldwork, when you intend to start the lab work and when you are aiming to finish. Obviously, some contingency should always be considered. The Gantt chart will help you secure funding since a sponsor may consider sponsoring you only if the delivery of the sponsored money is provided in instalments according to the Gantt chart. I had one of my main sponsorships actually follow such a procedure, where the allocated sponsorship of €50 K was divided into two instalments in accordance to the Gantt chart I prepared and presented.

Potential sponsors and funding opportunities will vary by region as well as by country. So, it is difficult to specify and list potential sponsors/funding opportunities. As a general rule, however, there are usually funding opportunities that are offered by the government or local organisations that you might be eligible for. Third parties such as foundations, banks, health insurances and pharmaceuticals are also potential sponsors. Nonetheless, when considering third parties as your sponsors, it is essential to ask upfront about their expected involvement in your research and any disclosures that might impinge on their sponsorship. If you are going to be sponsored from, let's say, a foundation that imports junk food, and they want to have access to and a say in your methodology, your results and conclusions, then there is a conflict of interest, especially if you are pursuing health-related PhD research. Such a conflict of interest may place your ability to publish your work in international journals at risk, and you may have to defend your choice of sponsors during your defence exam.

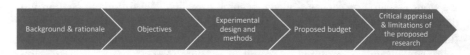

Fig. 3.2 Summary of the different sections of the grant proposal

Chapter 4
The Fieldwork

A PhD research study can follow different observational study designs. The most commonly used study design is a cross-sectional study that has a strong descriptive element. Through a *cross-sectional study,* information at one point in time can be collected including prevalence rates. It also provides analytical information through association studies between the outcome and potential exposures. This type of study design will be discussed later in further detail in this chapter. A *case-control study* is another study design that can be easily conducted as part of the design of PhD research. This type of study design explores the retrospective relationship between a disease cohort (the case) and a 'healthy' cohort (the controls). Ideally these cohorts are matched by age and sex for comparisons. However, both of these designs have their limitations. Both types of studies are unable to account for temporal relationships between the exposure and the outcome as well as being subject to selection bias.

Defining the Population

The first step in any epidemiological study is to identify the target population, i.e. the population you want to study. If we are to take an example from my own PhD, the target population was adults between the ages of 18 and 70 years who were residents in my country [1]. Next comes the population sampling. This will depend on whether you are aiming for a national/regional/state representation or you are going to investigate a particular group, e.g. school children in your local school district. Ideally a random process is followed to avoid selection bias, but it may not always be feasible, especially if you are going to investigate a minority group. In my case, since it was a national study, the aim was to have a sample population representing approximately 1% of each sex (Males and Females) living in each town and following within each age group. Considering that the main aim of the study was to explore

© The Author(s), under exclusive license to Springer Nature Switzerland AG 2021
S. Cuschieri, *To Do or Not to Do a PhD?*, SpringerBriefs in Public Health, https://doi.org/10.1007/978-3-030-64671-4_4

pre-diabetes and diabetes, the population sampling was based on the expected prevalence of pre-diabetes [1]. The PiFace® software, with a maximum confidence interval of ±5%, was used to estimate the required sample size of participants with pre-diabetes. From this estimated population sample (which was approximately 25% of the population), the required total sample population was estimated. However, it was anticipated that a 50% response rate would be achieved based on previous local studies; hence, the final sample population size needed to be double the amount that was calculated by PiFace® [1]. The next step is to run a random sampling procedure to obtain the actual sample population from a selected database. The random stratification can be either single-stage or two-stage sampling depending on the size of the country/region/state that you are examining. In my case, as my country has a small population size, a single-stage random stratification was performed. However, in larger countries or regions, a two-stage sampling is required to keep the survey geographically feasible. The latter sampling methodology would estimate a larger sample population than the former since two-stage sampling is subject to a design effect of 1.5 [2]. If you are currently confused by all these sampling technicalities, do not worry; speak with your supervisor or a statistician. Something to remember is to clearly establish the inclusion and exclusion criteria for your sample population, for example, pregnant women, people too sick to leave their homes and those living abroad even on a temporary basis were excluded from my PhD study.

Preparation for the Health Survey

There are two types of health surveys: (1) Health Interview Survey (HIS) and (2) Health Examination Survey (HES). The HIS is based on data collection through self-reported questionnaires that are either self-administered or interviewer-led. Such a survey is able to measure health status, health behaviours and history of known diseases. However, it is not able to provide any information on undiagnosed conditions or any factual measurements such as height and weight. This mode of data collection is subject to reporting bias.

The HES is composed of a health examination for different anthropometric and biochemical parameters such as blood pressure, waist circumference and drawing of blood samples. It is usually accompanied by a questionnaire for socio-demographic data and medical history.

Questionnaire

The questionnaire used for either a HIS or a HES needs to be validated; i.e. the questions need to have been proven to provide adequate information. There are a number of readily available validated questionnaires covering a range of health topics. Researchers can utilise these questionnaires provided that adequate acknowledgement or permissions are obtained. Examples of these validated questionnaires are: the demographic health survey (DHS) used to collect demographic data (https://dhsprogram.com); the World Health Organization (WHO) step-by-step risk surveillance of noncommunicable diseases (https://www.who.int/ncds/surveillance/steps/instrument/en/) and the WHO global adult tobacco survey (GATS) used to evaluate tobacco use (https://www.who.int/tobacco/surveillance/tqs/en/).

The mode of delivery for how these questionnaires are distributed to the study population can include postal mail, electronic mail, telephone interview or face-to-face interview. Based on my experience, I found that face-to-face interviews facilitated completion of questionnaires since the interviewer leads the session. I was lucky that I could afford to follow this mode of delivery. However, this is not always the case. Nowadays the extensive availability of online technology has made it a more feasible and acceptable mode of delivery. The choice of best delivery modality is up to you and the resources available to you.

Health Examination

A health examination provides you with the most accurate form of physical health information especially when assessing for undiagnosed conditions. Standardised physical health information protocols should be followed in order to be able to compare your results to other local or international studies. Validated tools of measure should be used. As an example, if a blood pressure monitor is going to be used, then it is essential to use a sphygmomanometer that has been proven to provide accurate results in surveys. There are also validating entities that will grade the instrument such as the 'Association for the Advancement of Medical Instrumentation' and the 'British Hypertension Society'.

Recruitment of Fieldworkers

You as the PhD student must be the prime fieldworker as this is your PhD after all. Alas, if the study you are conducting will require examining or interviewing a large number of participants, doing everything on your own may not be sustainable. Considering my case, where I had to contact 4000 adults with an expected 50% response, it was impossible to do all of the interviews, examinations and bloodletting on my own. I had to recruit a small number of fieldworkers who were willing to learn the study's protocol, undergo regular training sessions and work in a teamwork environment. If you are going to have someone helping you out, even if it is just one person, it is essential that the same protocol and techniques are followed in order to avoid interpersonal variations. Therefore, it is paramount that regular training and validation of your protocol and technique are performed. If you fail to have such a unified technique, your data will not be accurate, and you are open to criticism and difficulties in data interpretation and reporting.

Pilot Study

A pilot study is advisable to be conducted prior to every epidemiological study, to ensure that the protocol design is actually sustainable. Through a pilot study, you conduct your planned study on a smaller scale, so it is easier to identify any bottlenecks or problems. It is also the appropriate time for fieldworkers (if present) to practise in a controlled environment and try to reduce inter-observer bias. Some students may foresee the pilot study as a 'waste of time'. I did fall into this trap myself; however, with time I learnt that I was wrong. Through the pilot study I realised that the appointment schedule that I had planned was flawed. Appointments were too far apart and there was a lot of idle time between participants. Another lesson learnt was that the 'elderly' subgroup preferred an earlier appointment (6.30 am onwards), while the 'younger' subgroup appreciated later appointments (8 am onwards) [1, 3]. Something to keep in mind is that the participants who take part in the pilot study cannot be included as part of the actual study.

Setting Up Your Fieldwork

Whether you are following an interview-based study or a health examination study, you need to inform your participants about the study itself. The means of communication will vary by the type of study you are conducting. For example, if you are using online means for dissemination of an electronic questionnaire (provided that you have email addresses or other online platforms), then online communication is justified. Using this method automatically will limit participation to those having an internet connection and/or electronic mail account. Even in this era of high tech, not everyone can avail themselves of such an account, especially the elderly and individuals of low social economic status. It is therefore important to weigh your pros and cons when choosing your preferred method of dissemination. In my case, I was provided only with the home address of the random sample population. Therefore, I did not have much of a choice but to send out an invitation letter to their home address using traditional post. There are a lot of practical problems using this method. The letter can get lost, it gets thrown away immediately by the recipient, the participant moved houses and has not yet informed the authorities about it and some letters are returned to you. Having no other means of contact was frustrating since I was at the mercy of the potential participants to reach out to me. The invitation letter sent to the study population presented a detailed explanation of what the study consisted of, along with the benefits of their participation. Participants were given a personalised appointment date and time at their local town clinic. We chose to do the health examination in local town clinics in order to enhance participation and try to avoid as much as possible any commute to the examination hubs. It was anticipated that this would enhance response rate. Participants were asked to confirm, cancel or postpone their appointment through either telecommunication or electronic means. Those accepting to participate were advised to abstain from eating or drinking anything but water for at least 9 h prior to their appointment (since fasting blood glucose and lipid profile blood tests were going to be performed) and refrain from smoking and physical activity for at least an hour prior to the appointment. Confidentiality was assured, and they were informed that all of the measurements and results obtained would be communicated back to them. Those who confirmed their attendance were asked for their mobile number in order to send them a text appointment reminder a day prior to their set appointment date. This proved to be a very efficient way to achieve a good response rate [1, 3].

On the day of the examination, it is important to ensure that the person attending the appointment is the actual person who was invited to attend. If you are following a random selection of participants, it is important that only the individual who was randomly selected participates. Not even an identical twin is eligible! An informed consent is the next step. This will depend on the mode of delivery of your study. If you are using a telephone call to ask questions, then a verbal informed consent can be obtained; however, if you are using online communication or a face-to-face approach, then a written informed consent is a must. The next steps will vary according to the type of study you are conducting. In my case, the health examination was divided into different stations. The participants first had an interviewer-led validated questionnaire, which gave them time to relax and gain trust in us. This was followed by blood pressure measurements (while still sitting down after approximately 20 min of the questionnaire); weight, height, and waist and hip circumference were next to be measured. The last station was bloodletting before moving on to the farewell station, where I (as the medical doctor on site) gave the participants an explanation of all of the anthropometric measurements taken (they were also given a copy of these results). I further advised them that the blood results would be sent to their home address via post, but should there be any abnormality I would call them immediately [1]. This proved to be very well-accepted by the participants.

There are conflicting trains of thought on whether participants should be given a token of appreciation. Some may view this as a 'bribing' method while others consider this as an appreciative gesture. For my study, it was deemed appropriate to provide the participants with a small bottle of water and some vouchers (which were sponsored through retail shops without any conflicts of interest). We embraced a very strict policy that no monetary or any conflicting items (e.g. voucher for a fast food meal) would be provided to the participants.

Data input is another issue that needs to be considered. Again, this is dependent on the mode of delivery of your study and the budget available. If you are conducting an online study, then the participant does all the work himself/herself. However, you would still need to go over the responses either to code them into categorical codes (e.g. Yes = 1, No = 2) or to make sure that the responses are coherent. On the other hand, inputting data for telephone call and face-to-face studies can follow a two-fold procedure. Ideally all data is entered electronically immediately; however; such a method may not be sustainable. If you as the PhD student and conducting the study on your own, then using your personal laptop or tablet to input data into a pre-designed form could be feasible. This holds true as long as you ensure that all data is encrypted or stored in safe manner. However, such as in my case, with more than one fieldworker helping me out as well as multiple stations along with a low budget, data entry in an online form was not sustainable. Therefore, everything was noted in the questionnaire booklet that also had the back pages printed with the anthropo-metric measurements. The participant was asked to carry the booklet from one sta-tion to the other until the end, when the booklet was collected while a copy of the anthropometric parameters was provided to the participant. Nonetheless, this method led to the inconvenience of having someone input all the data into an elec-tronic form. Such a method is subject to inputting errors. Hence, in order to try to minimise this, the secure online form used was validated (i.e. drop-down selections or cut-off points were used) to try to reduce errors. Furthermore, every week ran-dom spot-checks were performed, in which random booklets were cross-referenced to the inputted data. I am happy to report that errors were never identified. This laborious job could have been avoided should every fieldworker had a tablet or a station with a laptop to input the data. Unfortunately, monetary constraints made this impossible in my case. As a note, when using online forms, it is essential that a secure form is used. Remember that you are storing sensitive data even if personal data is coded through a unique code.

Laboratory Fieldwork

Epidemiological studies also can take the form of laboratory fieldwork. A typical example is when trying to establish associations between a condition (e.g. type 2 diabetes) and a genetic mutation. There are various types of mutations as well as genetic techniques that can be followed, which are beyond the aim of this book. However, I will share some photos of different techniques that may be followed (Figs. 4.1, 4.2, 4.3, and 4.4).

Fig. 4.1 Putting samples in a centrifuge. This process is used to separate the serum from the rest of the blood components using a very high-speed process

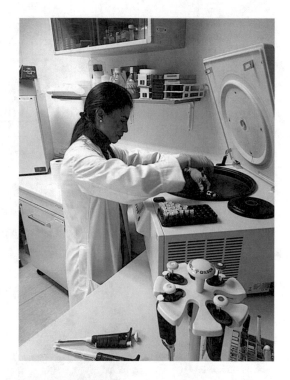

Fig. 4.2 Pipetting of aliquots is a very common technique used in every laboratory process. Different pipette sizes exist depending on the amount of aliquot you require

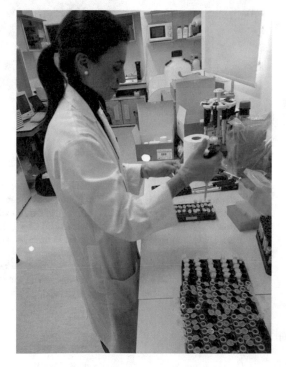

Fig. 4.3 A heat block is used to warm up the sample aliquots to denature the sample. The temperature is manually set. In this example, a 60 °C heat block was being used as part of a DNA extraction procedure

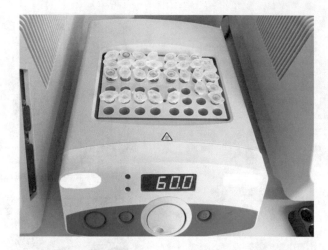

Fig. 4.4 A small centrifuge (**a**) is used to centrifuge a small number of samples for a short period of time using a constant speed. A vortex (**b**) is used to give a sample tube a quick mix

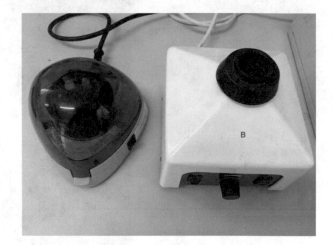

References

1. Cuschieri S, Vassallo J, Calleja N, Pace N, Mamo J (2016) Diabetes, pre-diabetes and their risk factors in Malta: a study profile of national cross-sectional prevalence study. Global Health, Epidemiology and Genomics 1:e21. https://doi.org/10.1017/gheg.2016.18
2. Axelson M, Sweden S-S, Bihler W, Bundesamt G-S, Djerf K, Lehtonen R, Agafitei L, Denisa E, Eurostat F, Gourdol A (2009) European Health Interview survey—Task Force III report on sampling issues. Eurostat European Commission p. 1–68
3. Cuschieri S, Mamo J (2020) Conducting a national representative cross-sectional study with limited resources: Lessons learned from a study in the small European State of Malta. SAGE Publications Ltd, 1 Oliver's Yard, 55 City Road, London EC1Y 1SP United Kingdom

Chapter 5
The Art of Data Analysis

I am not a medical or epidemiological statistician but rather a self-taught graduate making the best of online tutorials, asking experts and reading books and published articles to get through data analysis. In this chapter I give brief and simple explanations of the basic statistics that you will require for analysing your data originating from a cross-sectional study. I still recommend reverting to your supervisor or statistician to make sure that the analysis you have done is appropriate for your own study. In fact, my final analyses were reviewed by three independent advisors to make sure that the work was significant and correct.

The data you collect, either through an interview, examination or laboratory needs to be stored in one document. The easiest mode is by using a spreadsheet. Each participant should take up a row while the columns should represent the different variables that you have collected, which may range from age and sex to 'smoker or not', etc. Before trying to begin an analysis of any of your data, whether through a descriptive or an analytical modality or both, it is essential to standardise your data first. This means converting all data into numerical codes. This will help you analyse your data especially when using a statistical programme. There are a number of statistical programmes available but the most commonly used are either the IBM SPSS® or R® programme. I used the SPSS programme for my analyses. This section is based on this specific statistical programme.

Back to numerical codes: if the variable is a *continuous number*, e.g. age or 'number of cigarettes you smoke daily', then you have two options (both of which are important for your thesis): Option one: leave the number as it is, i.e. a continuous numerical variable. You will use this to calculate the mean/median or student t-test/Mann–Whitney-U test, etc. (to be discussed later). Option two: the continuous number is changed into a categorical range; this is usually performed using the statistical programme. In this scenario, the continuous data, e.g. age variable, is converted into, let us say, a 10-year age stratification, i.e. 10–19 years, etc. This will be used for descriptive, comparative and analytical work. Categorical data is also suitable for illustration of data through bar graphs. However, most variables will be

© The Author(s), under exclusive license to Springer Nature Switzerland AG 2021   29
S. Cuschieri, *To Do or Not to Do a PhD?*, SpringerBriefs in Public Health,
https://doi.org/10.1007/978-3-030-64671-4_5

Categorical variable		Numerical code
Smoking status	Yes	1
	No	2
Type 2 diabetes mellitus	Yes	1
	No	2

categorical in nature, e.g. highest education level, medical history, smoking or non-smoking, dietary habits, etc. In order to statistically analyse the categorical variables, it tends to be better if these are changed into numerical codes as seen in Table 5.1. It is essential that you keep a descriptive key or labelling of what each numerical code stands for.

A categorical variable can be sub-divided into two categories: (1) *Nominal*—where the variable in one category is no better than the other category, e.g. Smoking and Non-Smoking, Male or Female; and (2) *Ordinal*—where there is some order to the categories, e.g. highest education level. Such distinctions will be important depending on the statistical programme you use.

The Chi-squared test is the statistical test used to assess for any relationship between two categorical variables. However, if one variable is categorical and the other is continuous, the statistical test used will depend upon whether the data is parametric or not (to be discussed in the next section).

Parametric or Non-parametric?

The very first thing that you need to do is to establish whether the data you had collected follows a normal or a skewed distribution. This is essential since different statistical tests (for continuous variables) would be used in accordance with the type of data you have.

Normal distribution, also known as having a bell-shaped curve distribution, describes the distribution of the variables in a symmetrical order. In this symmetrical distribution, most observations will cluster around the central peak and the values further away from the mean will taper off equally in both directions. There are various statistical modes on how to establish the distribution of your data depending on the statistical programme at hand. In SPSS, the test for normality is performed through the 'Kolmogorov-Smirnov test', where the variables in question are inputted into this test algorithm, and the *p*-value obtained will determine if the variable is normally distributed (non-significant *p*-value) or skewed distribution (significant *p*-value) data. My PhD data was skewed, as seen in Table 5.2. Significant *p*-values were established through the Kolmogorov–Smirnov test.

When the data is normally distributed, then the mean is the appropriate test used to establish the average of the continuous variables. When comparing two means

Table 5.2 Kolmogorov–Smirnov test showing non-parametric data (Source: my PhD data results) [1]

| | Tests of normality | | |
| | Kolmogorov–Smirnov[a] | | |
	Statistic	df	Sig.
FBG (mmol/L)	0.241	1856	0.000
LDL (mmol/L)	0.036	1859	0.000
HDL (mmol/L)	0.065	1859	0.000
Triglycerides (mmol/L)	0.143	1857	0.000
Total cholesterol (mmol/L)	0.035	1859	0.000
Age	0.077	1861	0.000
BMI (kg/m²)	0.067	1861	0.000
Systolic Bp (mmHg)	0.075	1861	0.000
Diastolic Bp (mmol/L)	0.071	1861	0.000
Waist circumference (cm)	0.023	1861	0.023
WHR	0.472	1861	0.000

Table 5.3 Summary of parametric and non-parametric statistical testing

Comparison	Dependent variable	Independent variable	Parametric test	Non-parametric test
Two independent groups	Continuous	Categorical	Independent t-test	Mann–Whitney test
Paired groups	Continuous	Time variable	Paired t-test	Wilcoxon signed rank test
Three + independent groups	Continuous	Categorical	One-way ANOVA	Kruskal–Wallis test

originating from independent groups, then the 'independent t-test' is used. Meanwhile, if the means are paired (e.g. weight before and after diet), then the 'paired t-test' is used. Whether you use the independent or the paired t-test is dependent on your own data and goals. If you are going to statistically compare more than three means, then 'one-way ANOVA' would be required. These different statistical tests are called 'parametric tests'.

If your data is *skewed,* as was the case with my PhD data, then non-parametric tests are required. The median needs to be used instead of the mean. The median is the value sitting in the middle of a list of numbers. The 'Mann–Whitney test' is used to significantly compare two independent groups (continuous vs. categorical). On the other hand, when two groups are paired, the 'Wilcoxon signed rank test' is used. When more than three independent groups are compared, the 'Kruskal–Wallis test' is used. These tests are called '*non-parametric tests*'. Table 5.3 provides a summary of the parametric and non-parametric tests available and when they can be used.

When you have two continuous variables and you need to evaluate for a relationship between them, then for parametric data, the 'Pearson's r test' is used, while for non-parametric data the 'Spearman's rho test' is used. The 'R'/'RHO' score will determine whether the relationship is positive (upward slope) or negative (down-ward slope), while the p-value⁻ will determine whether the relationship is significant.

Descriptive Analysis

Descriptive statistics, as the name implies, will give a description or a summary of the features of your population. Common descriptive methodologies follow a per-centage, a prevalence, or a proportion of the population under study having a par-ticular feature. To measure the prevalence of a feature, e.g. type 2 diabetes, you need to know the number of cases (i.e. number with type 2 diabetes), divide this number by the total number of participants (study population) then multiply by 100. You can further stratify this data by sex, age groups, etc. This 'descriptive epidemiology' is used in epidemiology to describe the distribution of a disease and its determinants within the population. The disease frequency can be described in relation to geo-graphical area, education, etc. In order to establish whether your descriptions have any statistical significance, you will have to use the tests mentioned earlier in accor-dance with the type of data you are analysing, i.e. parametric or non-parametric and continuous or categorical data. Such analyses will provide what is called a 'univari-ant analysis'. There are several options on how to report the univariate data. This can range from a descriptive text to frequency distribution tables, bar charts or histograms.

Sometimes it is better to start off your analysis by 'eyeballing' the data. This means looking at the data set, descriptive tables or graphs available before carrying out any statistical calculations. By eyeballing the data, you may be able to identify trends or specific sequences that may catch your eye. These may be of interest or may add additional value to your results should you pursue them further. Eyeballing data does not mean a quick glance of the information. Rather, it means taking your time to roughly analyse the data before ploughing forward. Showing your data to your supervisor may be beneficial. This process may bring with it a number of debates between you and the supervisor, but PhD students can learn from the experience.

Analytic Studies

In epidemiology, analytic studies will enable you to test a hypothesis. If your data is originating from a cross-sectional study, then you can measure the association between a particular exposure and a disease. An example of a hypothesis: is increase in age associated with having type 2 diabetes? In such a case, you are analysing the relationship between two different variables. This can be called a 'bivariate analy-sis'. When a relationship between three or more variables needs to be explored, then a multivariate analysis will need to be conducted. Depending on your goals, there are many ways to perform this analysis. These analyses can vary from multiple regression analysis to factor analysis, additive tree, cluster analysis, etc. It is important to have a discussion with your supervisor about your goals and which analytical test(s) should be followed.

Reference

1. Cuschieri S (2019) The burden of type 2 diabetes mellitus, dysglycaemia and their co-determinants in the adult population of Malta. University of Malta

Chapter 6
Putting Pen to Paper to Publication

Acquiring the skill of scientific writing is a versatile and essential goal for a PhD student as well as a future academic or researcher. We are living in an era of 'publish or perish', where publishing scientific findings is a mandatory task faced by many for both personal success and future job prospects. As a PhD student, you are expected to try to publish at least one manuscript originating from your research (however, this expectation will vary by institution, so please acquaint yourself with your institution's specific requirements). If you are able to publish most of your results in peer-reviewed journals, it would be an added bonus for the final defence exam. When your manuscript has undergone rigorous peer review (usually from experts in the field) and is finally accepted for publication, such a process automatically validates your results and work. This will make it difficult for your future examiners to argue against the findings that you present.

Your initial task is establishing which of your results are 'publishable'. It is common knowledge that journal editors will consider manuscripts for their journal only if the manuscript submitted covers interesting or important findings. If you are curious about what editors look for in an article, have a read here: https://www.ncbi. nlm.nih.gov/pubmed/30578111. Negative results or common findings (e.g. the older you are, the higher the risk of developing diabetes) are usually frowned upon and rejected. On the other hand, interesting findings, unique findings or a hypothetical revelation are highly sought out. However, do not get frazzled if your findings do not fall under this category. Having a good grasp of what is publishable usually comes with experience (so speak with your supervisor for more information and guidance). It means you need to present 'common findings' in a manner that whet editors' appetites. It all depends on how you deliver the results, the way the manuscript is constructed and how fancy the title sounds.

It is quite common to have your first attempt turned down. No need to feel rejected, down in dumps or disheartened. Rather, dig deep in your character, learn from the reviewers' comments, from your own supervisor's advice and from published articles covering your area of research. Once you establish the aim and

© The Author(s), under exclusive license to Springer Nature Switzerland AG 2021 35
S. Cuschieri, *To Do or Not to Do a PhD?*, SpringerBriefs in Public Health,
https://doi.org/10.1007/978-3-030-64671-4_6

objectives of your manuscript, in other words, which part of your results you want to share with the scientific community, then you are ready to start structuring your scientific paper in a more targeted manner.

Structuring a Scientific Paper

A scientific paper is composed of a number of sections following a structured format. When you get to submit your finished manuscript to a journal, you will notice that each journal will have its own specifications (e.g. different referencing styles); however, the basic structured format is always the same.

1. *Title*: The title of your manuscript needs to be short, comprehensive and eye-catching. It needs to intrigue the editor and later on the readers to read your article. The title should contain the specific identifier that your manuscript will focus on; e.g. '*The epidemiology of type 2 diabetes*'. Sometimes it is also useful to add the type of study design your results are originating from; e.g. '*The epidemiology of type 2 diabetes—Results from a cross-sectional study*'. No abbreviations are permitted within the title.
2. *Abstract*: The next section is the abstract. This gives a summary of the results of your scientific paper. An abstract can make or break your paper, since most readers (including editors) will just read your abstract. If the abstract is well-written and impressive, then there is a high probability that the full article is read. The abstract word count will vary depending on the journal; however, it is usually between 150 and 300 words. If the word limit is exceeded, the abstract will be rejected. Since the abstract is a summary of the actual full article, it is usually structured into the same sub-sections as that of the full article; i.e. *Background or Introduction, Aim/objective, Methods, Results and Conclusion*. In order to adhere to the word limit, it is essential to list only the most paramount information in the different sections.
3. *Keywords*: It is customary for five or six keywords to be listed after the abstract. The keywords consist of one or two words that describe the article. These keywords are especially essential for indexing of articles in different databases (more details on indexing later on). In order to make sure you are providing appropriate keywords, the US Library of Medicine provides the tool 'MeSH on Demand' (https://meshb.nlm.nih.gov/MeSHonDemand) as well as 'Medical Subject Headings' (https://meshb.nlm.nih.gov/search) that can be used to identify acceptable scientific keywords.
4. *Introduction*: The first section of your full-text article is the introduction. The introduction sets the stage for what is to come, i.e. your study's aim, objectives and results. A summary of the current knowledge (literature review) on the subject needs to be provided while pointing out the potential gaps in knowledge that require further exploration (this needs to allude to what you have studied). Then you introduce a background of what hasn't been studied and what your study

aims to investigate. A clear scope, novelty and significance of the article needs to be provided. In a nutshell, the introduction needs to answer two basic questions: (1) 'What is the article about?' and (2) 'Why should the reader bother to read your article?' [1]. It is paramount that you do not plagiarise while writing your literature review [2].

5. *Methods*: This section needs to give a detailed account of the 'what' and the 'how' of the study you are presenting. Sufficient details should be provided to allow someone else to replicate the study [3]. Therefore, a description of the study population, definitions used, the procedures/protocol and statistical analyses need to be provided. You need to mention the statistical software that was used as well as report the permissions and ethical clearances that were obtained. Do not forget to list the inclusion and exclusion criteria that were followed. Depending on the research study design method you are describing, readily available international guidelines and checklists have been formulated and reported, as summarised in Table 6.1. It is recommended that you familiarise yourself with these guidelines and adhere to them when presenting your work.

6. *Results*: This is the section where you communicate your observations, facts, findings and measurements. A logical order of the results needs to be followed; e.g. from the most important to the least important facts or from the descriptive to the analytical results. Using tables or figures will enhance the delivery of the results, but it is important not to repeat what you are illustrating in the written text. As a rule of thumb, the text is used to describe limited data while illustrations (tables and figures) are used to describe copious amount of data, correlations or trends. It is essential to cite and reference the illustrations in the text, while providing a concise caption underneath or above the illustration. Hence, illustrations can be stand-alone sources of data [11]. Clear and defined formatting of the illustrations will help the reader understand the information that you are trying to portray [11].

7. *Discussion—Conclusion*: It is mandatory not to repeat the results in this section. This section is used to combine the introduction, your aim and objectives to your results while discussing and linking them together. Your findings need to be compared with previously published literature, while an explanation is provided of how your results vary from the literature. Avoid overstatements or strong statements (e.g. The findings prove…); be humble and only suggest or recommend.

Table 6.1 A comprehensive summary of the guidelines for scientific writing of the most common research study designs

Research study design	Guideline
Randomised control trial (RCT)	CONSORT statement [4–6]
Study protocols	SPIRIT [7]
Systematic reviews	PRISMA [8]
Observational studies (e.g. cross-sectional)	STROBE [1, 9]
Case reports	CARE [2]
Qualitative research	SRQR [10]

8. *Acknowledgments*: This is the section where you recognise 'silent partners' for their contributions. There are authors guidelines (The International Committee of Medical Journal Editors—ICMJE) that need to be adhered to. According to these guidelines, authorship is based on four criteria: (1) Substantial contributions to the conception or design of the work; or the acquisition, analysis, or interpretation of data for the work; (2) Drafting the work or revising it critically for important intellectual content; (3) Final approval of the version to be published; and (4) Agreement to be accountable for all aspects of the work in ensuring that questions related to the accuracy or integrity of any part of the work are appropriately investigated and resolved [12]. Contributors who do not qualify as authors should be mentioned under 'Acknowledgements'.

   Full details are available on the ICMJE website: http://www.icmje.org/recommendations/browse/roles-and-responsibilities/defining-the-role-of-authors-and-contributors.html.

9. *References*: This is a list of all of the literature sources that were used in the paper. A citation within the text needs to be done with the full reference found in this section. A number of different reference styles are available; however, the most common styles are Harvard (in-text citations include the author's surname) and Vancouver (in-text citations consists of a continuous Arabic numbering sequence). Each journal will have its own reference style, so it is essential to check the guidelines for authors so that you adhere to their style. Nowadays there are a number of bibliographic management software available either for free or with a fee. Universities tend to offer students access to one of the many bibliographic management software as part of their graduate perks. This tool is used to create personalised databases and cite articles while compiling a manuscript or a document including the thesis. Different management software tools (e.g. EndNote, RefWorks, Mendeley, Zotero) offer different functions, strengths and weaknesses. Ultimately they all have the same utility; i.e. to help you to cite and reference your text [13].

Targeting the Most Appropriate Journal

The first decision you are faced with is, '*In which type of journal do you need to publish in?*'. There are two major categories of published journals: (1) subscription-based, also referred to as traditional or hybrid journals, and (2) open access journals. There is considerable debate on the pros and cons of publishing in either type of publishing journal; for further reading: https://www.ncbi.nlm.nih.gov/pubmed/29499986. The crucial difference is that the latter type of journal requires the author to pay an article processing charge (APC), which can range from a few hundred dollars to a couple of thousand dollars to publish one article with open access. Some students are fortunate that their university will cover this expense, so that open access journals may be considered. There are universities, however, that bind students to publish their research with open access only, the reason being that through an open access publishing mode, the article will be freely available immediately after publication to anyone across the world. This is unlike the subscription-based publishing mode in which only the abstract would be freely available. Nevertheless, the author needs to be careful not to fall prey to the world of predatory open access journals.

The next decision is the type of article you are going to write and submit for publication. The different types of articles include original articles (this should be your prime aim), review articles (this may be part of your thesis's literature review), case studies (not every journal accept these), commentaries, editorials, letters to the editor, and rapid review, among others. At your level as a postgraduate student, the most common types of articles you should be aiming for are the 'original articles' and 'reviews'.

Once you know the type of article you are going to write, then you need to identify a suitable journal. There is a plethora of journals available, so you need to be extra careful about where you try to publish your work. You need to decide whether you are going to aim for a general or a specialised journal; e.g. a journal of public health, a journal of epidemiology or a journal of health promotion. The decision depends on whether your article will be of interest to a sub-section of the public health community or to any public health specialist. A way to identify a suitable journal is to match your article's keywords to other published articles in a particular journal. However, this process may be time-consuming. There are web-based tools that will aid you in the quest for the perfect journal. These will help you identify potential journals that have previously published articles similar to your own. When it comes to choosing the perfect journal, ideally the journal should be widely read and well known in your research field. It is important, also, to note whether the journal accepts the intended article type, especially if the article is a review or a case report.

Deciding between one journal and another may be challenging, especially if you are an early career researcher and new to the publishing game. It is essential to know that reputable journals are 'graded' by various types of metrics such as journal Impact Factor (IF). For more information about research metrics read: https://www.ncbi.nlm.nih.gov/pubmed/29402491. The journal impact factor takes into account the citation frequency of the articles that were published in that particular journal, usually over a two- or five-year period, and compares it with other journals within the same speciality. Although influential factors can affect this type of grading, it gives the author an indication of the journal's impact or quality within the specific scientific community, e.g. the international public health community. The higher the journal's impact factor, the more influential and prestigious the journal is. However, this also means that it is tougher to get an article published in such journals because they usually have a high rejection rate and low acceptance rate (10–20%). If your article is not reporting cutting-edge research findings, it might make sense to downscale to lower impact journals rather than high impact journals. You can still try your luck by submitting to a high impact journal. There is nothing to lose, but it means that most probably you are delaying the publishing process. Having said that, if your rejected article manages to go out for peer review, i.e. it is not rejected immediately at the editorial stage (the initial stage), you may get valuable feedback from different reviewers. Such constructive feedback will help you review your paper from the point of view of expert researchers in your public health field. It may be a rejection, but it will serve as a learning curve. The morale of the story is to never give up. You may need to tweak your article a couple of times, but if it is worthy research, you will get it published eventually.

Another factor an author tends to take into consideration is 'indexing'. I take indexing very seriously when choosing a journal. Indexing means that the journal in question would be featured in a number of different databases through which other researchers can find your article. There are a number of indexing databases available such as PubMed, Medline, Google scholar, EMBASE and SCOPUS, among others. Journals that are indexed in renowned databases reflect the quality of the journal. For example, for a journal to be indexed in PubMed and Medline, it needs to pass a long and rigorous review process. Personally, my gold-standard rule is that if the journal is indexed in either PubMed or Medline, then it is a good choice. It does not mean that I have never published in journals that are not indexed in these databases, because I have, but if I had the choice, I would opt for journals that are indexed in these databases.

These are the basic factors that should be considered when faced with the dilemma of which journal to choose. However, there are other factors that you may be interested to know; for further reading: https://www.ncbi.nlm.nih.gov/pubmed/30579738.

References

1. Cuschieri S (2019) The STROBE guidelines. Saudi J Anaesth 13:S31. https://doi.org/10.4103/SJA.SJA_543_18
2. Gagnier JJ, Kienle G, Altman DG, Moher D, Sox H, Riley D, the CARE Group (2013) The CARE guidelines: consensus-based clinical case reporting guideline development. Glob Adv Heal Med 2:38. https://doi.org/10.7453/GAHMJ.2013.008
3. Lin PY, Kuo YR (2012) A guide to write a scientific paper for new writers. Microsurgery 32:80–85
4. Moher D, Schulz KF, Altman DG, CONSORT (2001) The CONSORT statement: revised recommendations for improving the quality of reports of parallel group randomized trials. BMC Med Res Methodol 1:2. https://doi.org/10.1186/1471-2288-1-2
5. Moher D, Hopewell S, Schulz KF, Montori V, Gøtzsche PC, Devereaux PJ, Elbourne D, Egger M, Altman DG, Consolidated Standards of Reporting Trials Group (2010) CONSORT 2010 Explanation and Elaboration: updated guidelines for reporting parallel group randomised trials. J Clin Epidemiol 63:e1–e37. https://doi.org/10.1016/j.jclinepi.2010.03.004
6. Cuschieri (2019) The CONSORT statement. Saudi J Anaesth 13:27. https://doi.org/10.4103/SJA.SJA_559_18
7. Chan A-W, Tetzlaff JM, Altman DG, Laupacis A, Gøtzsche PC, Krleža-Jerić K, Hróbjartsson A, Mann H, Dickersin K, Berlin JA, Doré CJ, Parulekar WR, Summerskill WSM, Groves T, Schulz KF, Sox HC, Rockhold FW, Rennie D, Moher D (2013) SPIRIT 2013 statement: defining standard protocol items for clinical trials. Ann Intern Med 158:200. https://doi.org/10.7326/0003-4819-158-3-201302050-00583

8. Moher D, Liberati A, Tetzlaff J, Altman DG, PRISMA Group (2009) Preferred reporting items for systematic reviews and meta-analyses: the PRISMA statement. PLoS Med 6:e1000097. https://doi.org/10.1371/journal.pmed.1000097

9. von Elm E, Altman DG, Egger M, Pocock SJ, Gøtzsche PC, Vandenbroucke JP, Initiative STROBE (2007) Strengthening the Reporting of Observational Studies in Epidemiology (STROBE) statement: guidelines for reporting observational studies. BMJ 335:806–808. https://doi.org/10.1136/bmj.39335.541782.AD

10. O'Brien BC, Harris IB, Beckman TJ, Reed DA, Cook DA (2014) Standards for reporting qualitative research. Acad Med 89:1245–1251. https://doi.org/10.1097/ACM.0000000000000388

11. Cunningham SJ (2004) How to write a thesis. J Orthod 31:144–148. https://doi.org/10.1179/146531204225020445

12. ICMJE (2020) Recommendations | Defining the role of authors and contributors. ICMJE, http://www.icmje.org/recommendations/browse/roles-and-responsibilities/defining-the-role-of-authors-and-contributors.html. Accessed 15 Oct 2020

13. Cuschieri S, Grech V, Calleja N (2019) WASP (Write a Scientific Paper): the use of bibliographic management software. Early Hum Dev 128:118–119. https://doi.org/10.1016/j.earlhumdev.2018.09.012

Chapter 7
Writing the Thesis

The writing of a thesis is a requisite of the PhD you follow. A thesis is essentially a long essay describing the research conducted by a candidate for a university degree. Many students will see this task as potentially boring and daunting. True, there are more exciting things you can do instead of spending hours on end sitting down and writing. However, there is a silver lining to this task. Essentially, this is the last stage of your long PhD journey, so you can perceive the thesis as the last milestone to your 'freedom'. Furthermore, the skills that you develop during this PhD period will lay the foundations for your academic/research life that you may embark on in the future. On the bright side, thesis chapters can be substituted (with a little tweaking) into potentially publishable original or review articles. So, your efforts during the writing of the thesis will not be in vain.

Thesis vs. Research Manuscripts

A thesis and a research manuscript (as described in Chap. 6) have similar structural formats. A research manuscript aims to disseminate important or interesting findings established during the research study. A journal tends to restrict the word count limit for original research articles with a range of 2000 to 6000 words. On the other hand, a thesis is an academic document with the aim of addressing a hypothetical research question(s) with a higher maximum word count of usually around 100,000 words. The process leading to a thesis is laborious and follows a number of university regulations unlike that for a research manuscript. A research manuscript would entail choosing the ideal journal (as described in Chap. 6), after which all that is left is to make sure the structure or format of the manuscript abides by the guidelines for authors. Once that is done, you submit your manuscript and you are done. Both the thesis and the research manuscript need to be based on accurate referencing of the

© The Author(s), under exclusive license to Springer Nature Switzerland AG 2021   43
S. Cuschieri, *To Do or Not to Do a PhD?*, SpringerBriefs in Public Health,
https://doi.org/10.1007/978-3-030-64671-4_7

literature sources while avoiding plagiarism. Although a thesis is similar to a research manuscript, the journey is longer.

The Structure of a Thesis

The structure of a thesis usually follows similar sections like those of a research manuscript (as described in Chap. 6), i.e. Introduction, Methods, Results and Discussion. However, there are additional sections that need to be included in a thesis that typically are not part of a research manuscript; for further reading: https://pubmed.ncbi.nlm.nih.gov/30086984. The following list is the recommended thesis format advocated by many universities:

- Preface

  - Title page
  - Table of Contents
  - List of figures
  - List of tables
  - List of Abbreviations
  - Declarations
  - Acknowledgments
  - Abstract

- Introduction/Background
- Materials and Methods
- Results
- Discussion including study limitations
- Conclusion including recommendations
- References
- Appendices including any published articles from your PhD

The Title Page This should include the title of your thesis at the centre of the page. A couple of rows down you will write your name and any qualifications you have already achieved. The font size of your name needs to be one or two sizes smaller than that of the title. Next comes the name of your institution and the degree for which the thesis is being submitted, i.e. PhD. The next blank page needs to have the 'Declaration of Authenticity' statement. Here, you as the student declare that the work being presented in the thesis is your own original work and has been performed for the purposes and objectives of your PhD study.

The Table of Contents This consists of a list of the major thesis divisions along with their corresponding page numbers. It is customary that the page numbers of the sections before the 'Introduction' (i.e. the Preface sections) use Roman numerals (i.e. I, II, III), while from the 'Introduction' onwards, the pagination follows the

Arabic numeral system (i.e. 1, 2, 3, etc.). The table of contents does not usually have any page numbers.

List of Figures and List of Tables These two sections will include a list of the figures and tables (illustrations) that have been included throughout the thesis. In these sections, the Arabic-numbered Figure or Table along with the caption of the respective illustration and the corresponding page number are noted. Most writing software have the facility of creating the list of figures, list of tables and the table of contents automatically.

Acknowledgments Here you acknowledge all of the people involved in the research as well as those who have helped you in any way during this journey. This may include supervisors, co-supervisors, advisors, fellow colleagues, fieldworkers, etc. This is also the place where you show your gratitude towards your family and friends. They are usually embroiled in the emotional rollercoaster that you as a PhD student will experience.

Abstract This section is a summary of your thesis. It should give a background of the study, the objectives set, the basic methods, the important results and their associated conclusions under the different headings of: *Background, Aims, Methods, Results and Conclusion*. The word count for the thesis abstract is much more than that for an abstract of a research manuscript; however, every institution has its own guidelines. No citations are included in the abstract. In summary, the abstract should address the following questions: 'What was done?', 'Why was it done?', 'What questions were set to be answered?', 'How was it done?', 'What was learnt?', and 'Why does it matter?' [1].

Introduction or Background (Check with the University's Guidelines for the Appropriate Heading Title). This sets the scene for your thesis by providing a critical literature review of the topic you are investigating, e.g. type 2 diabetes. The introduction chapter needs to motivate and lure the reader into continuing to read your thesis by describing the problem at hand and the niche present in the scientific world that your thesis will address. It is paramount that the aim and objectives of the thesis are kept in mind while you are doing the literature review in order to stay on track and not deviate from the topic. All citations should originate from the original data source and not utilise other researchers' reviews and interpretations of the original research. Since this chapter is usually laid out during the initial phases of your PhD, it is important to keep updating the chapter with any new concepts, findings, studies and guidelines that may get published along your PhD journey. Personally, I suggest that you start this chapter early on. Most of the literature review is required as part of your PhD proposal, so once you already have laid the foundations, write it down in the form of an introduction chapter for your thesis. Having at least one chapter completed (even if you would need to update it along the way) means one less thing on your agenda when you reach the thesis-writing stage. It is recommended that the methodology you followed for your literature review is noted down;

i.e. the search strategy including the inclusion and exclusion criteria. Furthermore, in order to facilitate the reader's experience, subheadings should be used throughout the literature review chapter. The final section of the introduction should give an outline of the reasons why your research is required along with the hypothesis and research questions being posed by your study.

Materials and Methods   This section needs to thoroughly cover the 'what' and the 'how' of the research design study. The study's definitions, protocols, sampling and analytical data need to be sufficiently reported so that anyone wanting to reproduce the whole study can do so with ease. Therefore, for an epidemiological study it is essential to give a detailed description of the target population, the sample population and the study population. A detailed account of how the study population was achieved, whether it was nationally representative or not, needs to be clear. The inclusion and exclusion criteria considered in the research study, including the choice of study population (e.g. pregnant women were excluded), need to be clearly stated. You need to give an account of the materials (including questionnaire), equipment and definitions used as part of your study's protocol. This is followed by how you recruited your participants, trained your fieldworkers (if applicable) and where the fieldwork was conducted. A detailed account of all the permissions and ethical approval need to be present in this chapter as well. In other words, all of the preparations needed for the fieldwork need to be listed (as described in Chap. 4). Finally, all statistical analyses, calculations and calibration plots need to be noted down (as described in Chap. 5). All of this information must demonstrate your understanding of the methods required to address the hypothesis and research question(s) of your PhD. It is recommended that a number of subheadings are used such as:

- Subjects (*including target population, sample population, study population*)
- Design (*cross-sectional, case-control,* etc.)
- Definitions (e.g. *hypertension was defined as > 140 mmHg,* etc.)
- Materials, apparatus and procedure (*where applicable*; e.g. *questionnaire, weighing scales*, etc.)
- Statistical analysis (*parametric and non-parametric analysis, modelling,* etc.)
- Validity and reliability of method (e.g. *conduct of a pilot study*)
- Ethical considerations
- Permissions required

Results   This is the centre stage of your thesis, where you provide a clear interpretation of your research results. It must demonstrate your logic of inquiry while you were analysing your results data. All results, whether they are positive or negative, need to be reported.

Similar to a scientific manuscript (as described in Chap. 6), the use of tables and figures will enhance your presentation, provided these are clearly illustrated. It is important not to repeat results that are illustrated in a table or figure in the written text. As a rule of thumb, tables and figures are used to present a copious amount of information while text is used to describe limited data. When using tables or figures, avoid using a lot of colour combinations. It should be simple to interpret with a self-explanatory title (caption). The tables and figures need to have enough information and a good caption that can stand alone in a manner that a reviewer or examiner can easily comprehend the message you wanted to portray. The formatting of the tables and figures should be kept identical throughout the whole thesis. It is common practice in both thesis and research manuscripts that tables carry only horizontal borders and no vertical borders where possible.

You need to provide the p-value for any statistical analysis that was conducted regardless if portrayed in tables or figures or for in-text descriptions. The p-value is a statistical value that illustrates whether the null hypothesis is correct. The smaller the p-value, the stronger the evidence in favour of the alternative hypothesis. Usually a cut-off point of $p = <0.05$ is considered sufficiently strong for statistical significance.

The sequence of the results section should follow the same sequence as your methods. For example, initially if you described how the prevalence rate was calculated, then you moved on to how you compared the biochemical or anthropometric data by age, sex, etc., the results should follow suit. There is no definite sequence that should be followed (although check with your faculty in case there is an in-house regulation). If we take my own PhD results section [1], it was divided into five main sections (i) descriptive, (ii) analytic, (iii) association studies i.e. modelling (iv) a country specific diabetes risk score and (v) genetic studies, as below:

1. Descriptive analyses:

    (i)   Response rate.
    (ii) Age-sex profiles.
    (iii) Prevalence rates.
    (iv) Prevalence rates stratified by age groups and sex.
    (v)   Demographic characteristics (residential locality, education, employment) according to the general population and the different noncommunicable diseases under study.
    (vi) Lifestyle characteristics (smoking, alcohol habits and physical activity) according to the general population and the different noncommunicable diseases under study.
    (vii) Anthropometric characteristics (blood pressure profile, body mass index profile) according to the general population and the different noncommunicable diseases under study.
    (viii) Biochemical characteristics (lipid profile) according to the general population and the different noncommunicable diseases under study.
    (ix) Dysglycaemic population characteristics.
    (x)   Metabolic syndrome population characteristics.
    (xi) Depression population characteristics.

2. Analytic studies:

    (i)   Relationship between anthropometry, age and sex.

    (ii) Relationship between anthropometry and socio-demographic profiles.
    (iii) Relationship between anthropometry and lifestyle profiles.
    (iv) Relationship between body mass index, waist circumference and blood pressure.
    (v) Relationship between dysglycaemic population and anthropometry.
    (vi) Relationship between biochemical parameters, age and sex.
    (vii) Relationship between biochemical parameters and socio-demographic profile.
    (viii) Relationship between biochemical parameters and lifestyles.
    (ix) Relationship between biochemical parameters and body mass index.
    (x) Relationship between biochemical parameters and glucose regulation.

3. Association studies.
4. Diabetes risk score.
5. Genetic studies.

Discussion This is the section where you as a student 'shines' as you bring the theories behind your results to life. Here you discuss your findings and show the deep understanding of how your methods and results, along with your critical thinking, have evolved while comparing it to the published literature. When making comparisons with previously published studies, it is recommended that these studies would have followed a research methodology similar to your own. If you did a cross-sectional study, it is difficult to compare your results to a longitudinal cohort study since in the former no temporal relationships can be established unlike in the latter study design. If your results are contradicting the published literature, you need to carefully analyse them. If your workings and analyses are correct, it might signify a new finding that could change the way we think. Whatever the reason, you need to be able to justify or theorise the probable reason(s) behind your results outcome. Always be humble; you cannot discard other peoples' work as irrelevant. From personal experience, following the same sequence as that of your results will make your discussion read better. It is customary to include a section about your study's strengths and limitations at the end of the discussion. No study is perfect; again, you need to be humble in this section.

Conclusions and Recommendations In a public health PhD, this last section is crucial since here you are going to conclude your study, state what has been established and outline how this can be implemented for public health through policy or strategies. You should not repeat the results nor the discussion but rather note the take-home messages, as well as provide an interpretation of your results to be implemented at a population level. Remember, it is what public health is all about after all. As part of your recommendations, you may need to recommend further research in certain areas since as stated before there is no perfect study. All studies have their limitations.

References A list of all of the literature sources used within the thesis needs to be presented here. The sources may range from published articles (these should be your main sources) and guidelines to books and online websites (these should be reputable sources). Within the text, citations need to be provided and the whole reference needs to be written. There are various referencing styles, so it is important to refer to your institution's requirements, but the two major styles are 'Harvard' and 'Vancouver'.

The Harvard style consists of an in-text citation that includes the author surname(s), usually up to three authors, followed by '*et al*'. and the year of publication. Within the reference section, the whole reference is provided and arranged in alphabetical order by first author's surname.

On the other hand, in Vancouver style the in-text citation is an Arabic number. The numerical referencing sequence needs to illustrate the order each reference is used in the text. Later on, the same order needs to be followed in the reference section. The citation number used in the text either can be superscripted or within [square] brackets. The type of citation formatting needs to follow the institution's instructions.

As already discussed in Chap. 6, there are bibliographic management software programmes available either for free or for a fee that will aid you in referencing. These tools automatically cite and provide a corresponding reference list once you have uploaded or written the entire literature source. Universities tend to offer students access to one of the many bibliographic management software programmes as part of their graduate perks. There are different management software tools available (e.g. EndNote, RefWorks, Mendeley, Zotero), all with the same goal, i.e. to help you to accurately cite and reference your text.

Appendices The last section of your thesis hosts any additional data originating from your research that was not included in the results section but may be important for the examiner or anyone wishing to replicate the study. However, this is not the 'dumping area' for essential data that could not be placed in your results due to the word limit of the thesis. If you have published any parts of the thesis, this is the place where you provide a copy of your published articles.

Some ground rules when writing your thesis: First, plagiarism is a death sentence for you as it is a fraudulent manner of gaining academic recognition. Committing such a crime may result in your expulsion from the graduate system and bury any dreams of achieving the degree. So, if you want to use other people's work make sure you paraphrase and cite everything. At the end of your thesis period, you will be asked to upload the final version into plagiarism software that will determine whether you have copied any work. It is customary to upload a draft first so that you have an idea of where you stand and can amend any paragraphs that, even if they were paraphrased from the original source, may have matched someone's interpretation. A word of caution from my personal experience: If you manage to publish a large chunk of your thesis prior to the defence exam, it will help your case. The catch lies with the plagiarism software that may identify these parts as plagiarism. Even your own surname may be detected as plagiarism. So, it is important to: (1) try to paraphrase as much as you can when you publish your own work originating from the thesis, and (2) identify exactly what was highlighted as plagiarism and be ready to defend this in your defence exam.

Another rule to follow is that no footnotes are accepted in a scientific-based thesis. Anything you have paraphrased from published literature needs to be cited and referenced at the end of the thesis.

Finally, every faculty, institution and university will have its own regulations and styles for their students' theses. There may be variations in these regulations and styles even between faculties within the same university, so it is paramount that before you start writing your thesis, you identify and understand the exact regulations that your thesis needs to follow. This will save you a lot of headaches later on.

Reference

1. Cuschieri S (2019) The burden of type 2 diabetes mellitus, dysglycaemia and their co-determinants in the adult population of Malta. University of Malta.

Chapter 8
The Hurdles Along the Way: A Personal Experience

It is expected and inevitable to encounter hurdles and problems during the course of your PhD. These problems are multifaceted and usually crop up during different and least-expected situations. This is when resilience and hard grafting are essential.

You might encounter the first hurdle when you apply for a PhD programme. The actual process of putting pen to paper and submitting your PhD proposal might be stressful and unsuccessful in the first attempt. A rejection of the proposal by your first-choice institution is a common blow to one's expectations. This might feel like a punch in the gut, especially if you have been dreaming of becoming a graduate from a particular university for as long as you can remember. The next hurdle might arise when finding the right research question and niche to explore for your studies. Let's be realistic—science, epidemiology and public health have been around for decades, so finding an innovative niche might cause some head-scratching. However, if you are passionate about a particular topic, do not get frazzled. Think outside the box. What can you add to the area? Let's take myself, for example. I had finished both postgraduate and master's degrees in diabetes, seeing that it is my country's national disease. So for me, it was the perfect disease in which to invest. However, when it came to a PhD, I was faced with a brick wall because endless research has been done in this area. If digital health was my cup of tea, then that might have been a nice cosy niche. I don't consider myself an IT guru, so this idea had gone out of the window. It took several hours with several experts in the fields of epidemiology, public health and diabetology to come up with a significant title and research niche. I must admit that I was lucky to live in a country with a small population size and a lack of state resources to conduct research. Hence as a nation we were lacking recent public health data on our health status at a national level. This presented the perfect opportunity for my PhD to evolve and develop. As a general tip, it is essential that an intensive literature review is conducted. Assessing what other states, regions and countries have done and whether you can implement any of those ideas in your scenario is a great way to reach a desired research question. Also, discuss your idea(s) with colleagues or experts in the area. You never know who might give

© The Author(s), under exclusive license to Springer Nature Switzerland AG 2021   51
S. Cuschieri, *To Do or Not to Do a PhD?*, SpringerBriefs in Public Health,
https://doi.org/10.1007/978-3-030-64671-4_8

you a hint or an idea of what you can do. Obviously, if you are going to join a collaboration study as part of your PhD, then these problems are foregone.

Securing grants, scholarship and funding for your PhD is another headache. Students who are following a sponsored or scholarship PhD are usually exempted from such scenarios. This, however, is not across the board for all PhD students. I am one of the unfortunate ones. It took me almost 9 months of pestering different stakeholders to finally raise the required budget. My financial angels proved to be my university faculty, the research committee of the same university, another two major third-party stakeholders and other small donating stakeholders. They helped me raise over €100 K. If you are responsible for securing funding for your PhD, it is important to keep in mind the ethical implications of your funding source in relation to your PhD. When you are experiencing this stressful period, you might overlook some important disclosures that accompany your funding sources. A typical scenario would be securing funds from pharmaceutical or food and beverage companies when your PhD focuses on the health of a population, for example. You are in for an ethical conundrum. More and more so if your funding contract binds you to involve the funders in your study design or your analysis or data presentation. Remember that in order to publish your work, you need to disclose all of the funding bodies as well as any conflicts of interest. If such companies have been involved and had a say in your research, there is a chance that your manuscript might not be accepted for publication. However, this is not the only possible scenario that you might be faced with, since every case is different. So the moral of the story is, stop and think, evaluate and discuss with your advisors before accepting any funding.

Setting up your epidemiological fieldwork also might prove to be challenging. It all depends on your research design; however, each design has its own pros and cons. My study design was a cross-sectional health examination survey. A number of elements proved to be daunting. Setting up examination hubs with the required equipment in a different locality every weekend for a whole year was a logistical nightmare. This involved packing my 'Mary Poppins' car with all the equipment required including weighing scales, stethoscopes, bloodletting apparatus and questionnaires; obtaining the peripheral clinic key from health centres every Friday; and setting up the place in preparation for the weekend fieldwork. This included waking up early every weekend to be set and be ready for the first appointments at 7 am on Saturday and Sunday. On-the-spot decisions and adjustments had to be taken. Typically when participants did not turn up for their appointment even if they called to confirm their attendance, while others turned up with the invitation letter without previously confirming, the race against time was ever-present in order to transport the blood samples within the two-hour mark to prevent the samples from becoming haemolysed.

Another aspect is when laboratory work is required for the project at hand. Essentially, you need to learn the laboratory procedure including how to handle the pipettes and 96-well plates and how to operate the different laboratory apparatus such as autoclaves and centrifuges. Undergoing laboratory testing is a laborious procedure that requires extreme focus and diligence. There are various protocol booklets available to help the student perform a particular procedure, including instruction booklets offered by the manufacturers' kits should a student require laboratory or genetic kits. There is a definite learning curve in order to sharpen these skills. It is easy for a student to miss a step or contaminate a sample or else be faced with a stubborn test that refuses to obey orders even if the correct steps have been followed to the letter. As part of my PhD I had to extract DNA from whole blood by using specific kits and then undergo real-time PCR and genotyping, a process that took months to finish completely. A number of challenges presented along the way. Purchasing the required kits, apparatus, probes and chemicals through a draconian requisition system was my first challenge. I had to learn how to place a requisition and get quotes from different suppliers. Next was the adjudication process, followed by making sure to order the required items in the correct quantities. Delivery times and storage in the right conditions was the next issue. Having set all these in place, halfway through the DNA extraction process, it was noticed that a lot of the DNA extraction samples were impure. The most likely cause was established to be the DNA extraction kit that I was using. At the time, I felt like my world had suddenly collapsed since I had to abandon weeks of work and start all over again using a new DNA extraction kit. This, by default, necessitated the whole cascade described earlier, from purchasing to repeating the DNA extraction. Following this, a dramatic realisation dawned on me. Some participants' blood samples were running low because during bloodletting, only a small sample had been drawn. This piled on extra pressure in making sure that the second run of the DNA extraction ran successfully without further hiccups. When it came to PCR, this involved even more precision because I was working with micro-units and pipetting in very small 96-well plates. A small mistake would result in starting the process all over again for all 96 cases.

There are various rumours regarding PhD students vindicating their peers by knocking over their elbows while pipetting, resulting in the student losing hours of work. It is very heart-breaking to hear such disrespectful episodes of selfish human behaviour. I have even come across reports where students (especially females) are requested to share their collected blood samples with other PhD students in order for the latter to fulfil the PhD requirements, without proper consent or collaboration agreements. This is obviously unethical and should never happen. Collaborations between PhD students are essential when exploring a multifactorial subject such as type 2 diabetes. Such collaborations should enable more extensive research and output due to an increase in manpower and techniques. However, collaborations should be sought out and any creases in the agreements ironed out before the actual project commencement. It is unethical and abusive for students to share data with undisclosed 'colleagues' after succumbing to external pressure from more senior advisors, even more so when there might be an element of a gender issue.

During the course of the PhD, the student is at times in a psychologically vulnerable period. Hence, certain encounters with faculty members might be perceived as 'psychological abuse' especially if the topic at hand is close to the student's heart. Female students tend to experience such vulnerability states more frequently, especially when dealing with same-sex faculty members. It is important for the student to try to understand the argument at hand and consider the next move wisely. Making hasty decisions at the spur of the moment usually do not end well, even if you have been shouted at, felt belittled or treated unfairly. You need to be streetwise and stay focused on the end target. As a student, you have to accept your limitations and absorb any valuable advice. You cannot afford to irk your superiors by playing as a 'know-it-all'; remember, you are the student, and you need your superiors to sign off on your research and approve your final request to have your PhD thesis examined. There will always be a valid reason as to why you experienced such an encounter. Sometimes it may not be directly your fault but rather the circumstance you are in that resulted in such an encounter. Unfortunately, it is not uncommon to have multiple advisors who give conflicting advice on certain aspects of your research. It is a very uncomfortable situation to be in, especially when you are already stressed out. A helpful tip is that you seek guidance from an independent person, should you feel that the situation is getting out of hand. However, patience is a virtue that you need to learn as a PhD student. Sometimes, you may have to wait for a couple of days or weeks to get a reply. This does not mean that the person on the other end did not get your message or is disregarding your request. Most often it simply means that the other end has other, more urgent deadlines to meet.

Another point to keep in mind is that sacrifices need to be made during your research. Your life will change, and you are faced with deadlines, tough choices and decisions. During my genetic laboratory work I had to make a number of sacrifices. I used to arrive at the lab at around 6 am and keep on working until around 8 pm, irrespective of weekends and holidays. I remember myself at the lab, alone on Easter Sunday, dreaming about my customary Easter egg!! The reason for this tight deadline was due to a laboratory shift that I became aware of about halfway through my laboratory work. The equipment was going to be transported from the old laboratory to a new laboratory. Such a move meant that the PCR machine I was using would lose the present calibration, resulting in possible non-comparable results obtained pre- and post-relocation. Big red alarm bells went off in my mind. As a result, I needed to wrap up the PCR work before the move.

As already pointed out, each PhD journey is unique. Stress is a common denominator. Gender discrimination, intersectional hardships or any other form of racial, religious or social discrimination should never compound this. The student should be courageous and brave to stand for what is right and report any form of misbehaviour. Every institution has measures in place to help out students in such deplorable situations. Specifically, in cases of female students who get pregnant during the course of their studies, there should be measures in place to facilitate the ongoing project rather than pile on the pressure to keep to the deadlines. These might include temporary suspension of the studies without impacting the final outcome. It could be a rough ride but in the end, it will double the reward—PhD and your own child!!

The most important thing, although it is easier said than done, is for the student to be strong and never give up. It is the key to success. Unless one is psychologically and physically ready for such hardship, one may need to reconsider embarking on a PhD journey. We are all human, and at some point we all reach a breaking point. This is the point when family and friends (hopefully) step in and support you. But ultimately it is the student's stamina not to give up and to keep on fighting that will prevail in the end.

Chapter 9
Getting Ready for the Oral Defence

The PhD oral defence is the last step in your long PhD journey. Defending your thesis in-person in front of a panel of experts is the last essential stumbling block every doctoral researcher needs to surmount. The process from the thesis submission for examination to the actual oral defence date will vary from one university to another; however, the basis of this ritual is the same. It is essential to familiarise yourself with the oral defence process so that you can prepare adequately for the big day. Some universities, such as mine, require the student to prepare a 30-min presentation of their work before the actual interview exam kicks off. There are instances where the examiners decide to ask their questions during the presentation. So, be ready for everything. The duration of the oral defence will vary, typically lasting two to 4 h. You might be offered the opportunity to suggest whom you would prefer on your examining panel; however, not everyone will have that opportunity. I did submit my preferences, but the final approved examiners were slightly different from the suggested ones.

The main aim of the oral defence is to discuss your work in an interview-style exam with at least two examiners (internal and external). The number of examiners and spectators will vary by university. In my case, I had three internal examiners, one of whom was the chairman, and two external examiners. I also invited my supervisor to be a 'silent' spectator. Your examiners are experts on your subject field (e.g. diabetes), although no one will be an expert on your PhD work as much as yourself! If you have done all of your thesis work, then you know the nitty gritty of every step, every heartache, every failure and every success. It is what they will be looking for. If your thesis touches upon a number of different fields, you most likely will face examiners who are experts in the various fields. In my case, there were two epidemiologists, a diabetologist, a geneticist and a mathematical statistician. The examiners' main objective is to ascertain that you have 'gotten your hands dirty' with your data collection, analyses and writing of the thesis. They also are there to assist you with improving your argument for your thesis and possibly publishing your work. Another aspect that they will want to know is what you intend to do after

© The Author(s), under exclusive license to Springer Nature Switzerland AG 2021
S. Cuschieri, *To Do or Not to Do a PhD?*, SpringerBriefs in Public Health, https://doi.org/10.1007/978-3-030-64671-4_9

the PhD is over. Are you going to continue researching in the field or do you have other plans?

Preparing for the Big Day

The main focus of the oral defence is your thesis. It is imperative that you know it inside out. Reading and re-reading it is essential. Do not be alarmed if every time you do, you find a spelling mistake you had missed so many times over or a statistical working that is not correct. That is exactly what happened to me. I must have read it a hundred times over, along with my supervisor and my husband, but still I managed to fish out spelling mistakes as well as a crucial error in my statistics. Just a week before my oral defence, I realised that I had correlated categorical variables by mistake, when we all know that correlations can only be done for continuous variables. You can imagine my panic and worry at the time. I informed my supervisor about the problem, but there was nothing to do about it except wait for the day and confess my mistake. I was advised to own up to it if an examiner were to ask about it, which obviously was what happened. The mathematical statistician picked up the error. When it was his turn to ask questions, he brought it up for discussion. I apologised immediately. I explained that I had noticed it just a few days previously and had already amended it within the thesis, but it was too late to send an amended version of the thesis to all of the examiners. Being honest and owning up to my mistake resulted in a good outcome because the examiners were satisfied with my explanations and the interview moved on. The moral of the story is, know your thesis well and be humble and honest.

While reading through your thesis try to anticipate questions that may arise from each section. Know exactly how each section was carried out, the statistical analyses tests used and what could have been done differently. You are allowed to take a copy of the thesis with you; it is actually advisable to do so. Hence, I found it useful to write small notes on the thesis so that I could refer back to them should the need arise. It is paramount that the thesis copy that you provide to your examiners is the same as yours. Examiners may ask questions referring to specific pages during the exam, so it is essential that the page numbers and text match yours.

A number of standard questions may be asked during your oral defence, all of which will be structured and adapted to your thesis. The following are some typical questions that you may be asked:

1. Can you summarise your thesis?
2. What is the idea that binds your thesis together?
3. What inspired and motivated you to carry out this research?
4. Are there any current issues in the discussed field of study?
5. Why was the subject tackled and was it worth the effort?

6. Is there any work which is closest to yours? How does it differ?
7. What do you know about the history of your research question?
8. What crucial research decisions did you make?
9. Why did you choose this particular research design?
10. How did you deal with the ethical implications?
11. How have you evaluated your work?
12. Has your personal view on your research subject changed over the period of the PhD?
13. How do you know that your findings are correct?
14. What are the strengths and limitations of your work?
15. How could you have improved your work?
16. Who will be most interested in your work?
17. Summarise your key findings.
18. How do your findings relate to other literature in your subject field?
19. Does your thesis contribute to further knowledge in the subject field?
20. What have you learnt from the process of your PhD?

Although these are potential questions, you need to be prepared to adjust to what the examiners might ask you. If you are taken by surprise on a particular topic, don't dig your own grave. Admit your shortcomings and stay strong. Do not try to wing it as it may spiral downwards into a horrible experience. The same scenario also may occur if you go beyond what you have been asked for. Do not try to impress your examiners; just be true to yourself, stick to the point and you will not fail.

Another important point to keep in mind is your outfit for the day. It is advisable that you adhere to an interview etiquette, which is smart but most importantly comfortable. Do not wear something that makes you feel uncomfortable since it will hinder your performance. This also applies for shoes; do not wear a brandnew set of shoes for the day, especially if you think they may be uncomfortable in their first run. If you tend to sweat a lot during stressful periods, or feel hot or cold, make sure that your dress attire accounts for this. Personally, I know that I sweat when under stress, but I can feel very cold, as well, especially when there is air conditioning. Considering that my exam was in the summer, I decided to wear a dark dress with a light cardigan on top. This avoided embarrassing scenarios during the interview. The cardigan came in handy midway through the viva as I was getting increasingly cold. This way, I was dressed smartly and comfortable as well.

Asking your supervisor(s) for a mock exam is another important step in your preparations. Having someone 'grilling' you and putting you on the spot with potential questions is a much better trial than if you were to practise in front of your favourite teddy bear or while looking in the mirror, although the latter option is a good way to practise talking aloud.

It is also important to take care of yourself. Eating healthy food, remaining physically active and sleeping well are all essential factors that are required for success.

Preparing for Your Examiners

You will be informed of who your examiners will be prior to the oral defence. This information is usually contained in the same official letter that invites you to the oral defence appointment. Your job is to familiarise yourself with the examiners' work and research interests. Knowing how they think and what they like will help you prepare for your interview questions. Examiners will ask questions based on topics they know and potentially love. If they have published any articles that cover aspects of your research, I suggest that you read them well and familiarise yourself with the methodology and their results. I feel blessed that I did read a particular article that was supervised by one of my examiners since at one point my oral defence was directed towards this particular publication. If I had not read it, the outcome might have been painful and stressful for me. However, since I was well aware of the manuscript at hand, I could discuss the differences between my findings and those of the published article with ease. It also showed the examiners that I thought outside the box while preparing for the exam and I understood critical appraisal of other work.

After the Oral Defence

Just after the exam is over, examiners usually take a few minutes alone to discuss your performance before they call you back into the examination room. This may vary between universities. Those minutes of pacing and waiting behind closed doors were like a ticking time bomb for me. However, entering the examination room again and seeing smiles on the examiners' faces brought me relief. The chairman explained that there were some minor changes that needed to be addressed before the final thesis could be submitted officially and the journey ended. This was followed by a lot of congratulations and the opening of a bottle of champagne, a memory I will treasure forever.

It is the norm that you will have corrections following the oral defence. After the exam, the examiners will hand a joint report to the student that stipulates the corrections that are required. These may be minor or major revisions, also referred to as 'Re-submission'. The timeline to finish them varies depending on the extent of the revisions. Unfortunately, there may be instances where the outcome is not a happy one. Examiners may feel that the student did not reach the potential of a PhD level and may ask for revamped sections of the thesis, such as changing data analyses or discussion. The student may be asked to further the data collection. This may even mean that the student will not be eligible to graduate in that academic year with a possibility to participate in yet another oral defence examination. Different cases will have different outcomes and expectations. Nonetheless, failure of the PhD student is not the norm, so do not assume that you will experience this. As long as you do your part and prepare yourself, it will be a (stressful) walk in the park with a positive outcome at the end.

Chapter 10
What Comes After the Completion of a PhD?

Once the PhD journey comes to an end, it will feel surreal. You have been so focused, endlessly working hard for a number of years, and then all of a sudden you end up in a void, with no direct target in front on you. As you look at your hardbound thesis, with its sleek black leather cover and your name embossed shining in gold, reality will hit you. The PhD journey is over! What is next? Public health PhD graduates will have different aspirations and future plans. Some may take a year off to enjoy the fruits of the completion of the PhD by taking a break, maybe go on vacation (unless a pandemic hits, like COVID-19, and you are stuck at home in lockdown!). Others may have different plans or ambitions. Achieving the highest educational degree in the country doesn't necessarily equate to instant monetary rewards. The salary of an early career professional (post-PhD) is usually low. There always will be an income disparity between junior and senior professionals in any field. It need not frazzle you nor encourage you to burn any bridges. It should simply act as an incentive to keep working hard.

One can broadly divide the potential career opportunities into three categories: (1) academia, (2) government/public sector and (3) private sector.

Academia

One already may have a contract with a university as a research officer or a lecturer (assistant professor in the United States), which is part and parcel of the PhD contract. Those heading along this route already have an established opportunity in the (near) future, but others will not and may feel lost and uncertain about what to do next. If your interest is to follow the academic/researcher career path, then your next task is to be on the lookout for job opportunities at a university or an institute. For those wishing to pursue an academic/research path, a post-doctoral fellowship is highly recommended. A postdoctoral fellowship or postdoctoral research

© The Author(s), under exclusive license to Springer Nature Switzerland AG 2021
S. Cuschieri, *To Do or Not to Do a PhD?*, SpringerBriefs in Public Health, https://doi.org/10.1007/978-3-030-64671-4_10

experience is helpful but not an essential requirement. Undergoing such an experience enhances one's competencies as faculty personnel. The fellowship is a finite period of supervised training or mentorship that helps acquire and sharpen the skills necessary for your chosen career path. The application for a fellowship can be within the same university where you had conducted your PhD (if they offer such a programme) or at other universities or institutes. Such an appointment may be called 'postdoctoral research fellow', 'postdoctoral research associate' or 'postdoctoral research assistant'. If you are going to apply for a postdoctoral fellowship, make sure that it follows your professional interests such as population health, etc.

Organisations such as the World Health Organization (https://www.who.int/westernpacific/about/careers/fellowships) and the Centers for Disease Control and Prevention (https://www.cdc.gov/fellowships/full-time/doctoral.html) offer postdoctoral fellowships as well. Postdocs are often offered a temporary academic appointment during the period of their fellowship and this will enable the funding of the postdoctoral research. Others may have an appointment with a stipend or a sponsorship award. The postdoctoral position may be in preparation for an academic faculty position, although this is not always the case. During this period, it is expected that you produce a number of academic articles that are published in peer-reviewed journals or conferences.

Most universities in the United States, Canada and even in Europe (Sweden, Italy, Denmark, Germany, Finland, Belgium, Switzerland and The Netherlands) follow a tenure-track system, where an assistant professor (equivalent to senior lecturer) becomes an associate professor and then a professor. Usually an assistant professorship is the entry level in this tenure-track position system. A tenure grants the professor working at a university, permanent employment and a protection system from being fired without causation. This is close to 'academic freedom', which allows the professor to teach and research on any topic even if controversial. Those professors following a tenure-track appointment will need to undergo a tenure review every 6 years. During this tenure review, the professor's contributions to research, teaching and service to the university are evaluated through a dossier presented by the professor.

Public and Private Sectors

If your aspiration is to have an influential job in the policy-making positions of your country/state/region, for example, then you may consider a public/governmental position. Such positions may not be readily available at the time you finish your PhD, but it is always good to keep tabs on such openings and other related roles that eventually may provide you with the opportunity that you desire. Sometimes it may be more financially friendly to have an academic job in, let's say, the 'department of health services and policy' and wait on the sidelines. When there is an opportunity up for grabs in a governmental institute, you then apply already having gathered valuable work experience. Every country/state/region has its own system, so it is important for you to familiarise yourself with the respective system and be on the lookout. The take-home message is, do not give up. You may need to do another related or not-so-related job before you get to your dream job, but with determination and hard work you will get there.

Another potential field that a PhD graduate can aspire to is private-sector work. This may vary depending on your country or state. An example is working with an organisation such as the World Health Organization, which offers initial internships that might lead you to a permanent job. A word of advice: seeking such jobs may take you away from your own country depending on the location of the office of operations of the said organisation, unless you are offered a job that can be fulfilled by working remotely. These jobs may be harder to come by, but you can always keep tabs on their official websites or else look out for announcements they usually place in newsletters of public health associations.

Personal Experience

I consider myself lucky in this regard. I had a probationary full-time faculty position in conjunction with my part-time PhD studies. This automatically became a permanent one as soon as I achieved this degree. After completing my minor amendments and submitting my PhD thesis, I was at a bit of a loss. It felt strange not to feel a constant invisible pressure on my shoulders. My immediate post-PhD experience was very good, and I will cherish it for life, especially since just 5 months after finishing my PhD, the COVID-19 pandemic hit my country and I was forced to stay at home working remotely.

But that was not the end of my freshly minted post-PhD period. If you are determined to work hard and proceed with your professional life, there is nothing to keep you from doing that, not even a pandemic. Work-life balance is important as well as open communication with your partner (if you have one). Your professional life is important but so is your personal one, so do not bulldoze through to achieve your professional goal without considering your partner. Having said that, you still need to dedicate some time and work to put down roots in the academic/research world if you want to excel in your professional life. So, while I was still in the preparatory phase for my oral defence, I submitted a number of abstracts originating from my research (but not already published) to an upcoming European Public Health conference. I also applied to join a European health networking group covering an epidemiological concept that was new for me. I am always open to learn more, and this was a fantastic opportunity. Fortunately, both my abstracts and my application to join the networking group were accepted. Hence, just after my oral defence, I was on my way to an introductory meeting of the health network that served as a good stepping stone into the European epidemiological world as well as a networking experience. I made acquaintances with prominent epidemiologists in the subject field and I was also offered a short-term academic period at one of the expert's institutes to enable me to understand and work on this epidemiological subject. I welcomed this invitation with open arms, and it was a great and productive experience. This also led to collaborations with other European professionals that materialised into publishable articles in peer-reviewed journals. Attending the aforementioned conference also led to a great networking exercise.

One of my great ambitions actually was to write this book you have been reading for the past ten chapters. As a public health PhD student, I never found a concise book to read and help me through the PhD journey. I hope I managed to achieve my goal. So, while locked down at home during the COVID-19 pandemic, apart from delivering remote lectures and preparing examinations, I was working on research articles, some of which originated from my networking collaborators, some on COVID-19 (it was the season for it!) and some from my PhD dataset. I was also given the opportunity to contribute to chapters to three upcoming books that are going to be published by world-renowned publishers on subjects that fall under my research areas. If you are asking how I, a young career doctor, was approached out of all the global scholars, the answer is simple: I have published a number of articles in peer-reviewed journals that also have been cited a number of times as well as are accessible through well-known databases. Editors of books will search for 'experts' in the field by conducting a search of databases for authors who have published articles on the subject of the upcoming book.

It was beyond my wildest expectations that in less than a year of finishing my PhD I was able to accomplish so much, even in the midst of a pandemic. The key to success is networking and making international acquaintances, but at the same time remaining true to yourself. Whenever I got stuck, I acknowledged it and asked for help. Just because you have your PhD does not mean you know it all. There are always people out there to help you. It may be an old colleague of yours or a new acquaintance. Never be afraid to reach out and explore new opportunities. However, do not expect monetary payment for all of your academic efforts. Building bridges and publishing material will be your down payment, all of which will pay off at a later stage in your professional life.

The PhD journey can be seen as a daunting path. Some may think they are not worthy of it while others may think it is a piece of cake. Anyone who is determined and does not back out at the sight of a minor hiccup can apply for this qualification. The journey will not be easy, but if you believe in yourself and do your work, you can do it. Do not feel ashamed when you need to ask for advice or help. If someone closes the door on you, stop, think and see who else may be able to help you. Sometimes the most unexpected person may be your biggest supporter. The final result is worth all the hassles and heartbreaks. Achieving your Public Health PhD will open a world of many potential opportunities for you. It is, however, up to you to pursue these opportunities and your dreams. Never give up—you can do anything you set your mind to do.

Index

© The Author(s), under exclusive license to Springer Nature Switzerland AG 2021
S. Cuschieri, *To Do or Not to Do a PhD?*, SpringerBriefs in Public Health,
https://doi.org/10.1007/978-3-030-64671-4

Printed in the United States
By Bookmasters